MIDWIFERY PRACTICE

Postnatal Care
A research based approach

Edited by

Jo Alexander, Valerie Levy
and *Sarah Roch*

M
MACMILLAN

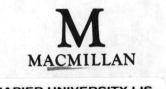

First published 1990 by
THE MACMILLAN PRESS LTD
Houndmills, Basingstoke, Hampshire RG21 2XS
and London
Companies and representatives
throughout the world

ISBN 0–333–53863–3 hardcover
ISBN 0–333–51371–1 paperback

A catalogue record for this book is available
from the British Library.

Printed in Hong Kong

Reprinted 1991 (twice), 1992

Contents

Other volumes in the Midwifery Practice series

■ **Antenatal Care**   ISBN 0–333–51369–X (paperback)
                        ISBN 0–333–53861–7 (hardcover)

1. *Joyce Shorney*: Preconception care: the embryo of health promotion
2. *Rosemary Currell*: The organisation of midwifery care
3. *Rosemary C. Methven*: The antenatal booking interview
4. *Jo Alexander*: Antenatal preparation of the breasts for breastfeeding
5. *Moira Plant*: Maternal alcohol and tobacco use during pregnancy
6. *Tricia Murphy-Black*: Antenatal education
7. *Jean Proud*: Ultrasound: the midwife's role
8. *Margaret Adams and Joyce Prince*: The psychology of pregnancy
9. *Jane Spillman*: Multiple births – parents' anxieties and the realities

■ **Intrapartum care**   ISBN 0–333–51370–3 (paperback)
                          ISBN 0–333–53862–5 (hardcover)

1. *Rona Campbell*: The place of birth
2. *Sheila Drayton*: Midwifery care in the first stage of labour
3. *Christine Henderson*: Artificial rupture of the membranes
4. *Judith Grant*: Nutrition and hydration in labour
5. *Alison M. Heywood and Elaine Ho*: Pain relief in midwifery
6. *Jennifer Sleep*: Spontaneous delivery
7. *Valerie Levy*: The midwife's management of the third stage of labour
8. *Carolyn Roth and Janette Brierley*: HIV infection – a midwifery perspective

Contributors to this volume

Margaret E Adams MSc SRN SCM MTD DN
Queen Charlotte's College of Health Care Studies, London.
As an experienced midwife teacher, Margaret Adams' interests are wide, but, in particular, she regards the development of interpersonal skills as a priority for midwives. She has written on midwives' styles of communication in the second stage of labour as part of a master's degree in social research methods.

Jenifer M Holden MPhil (Edin) BSc (Hons) Psychology SRN HVCert
Research Associate, Nursing Research Unit, Department of Nursing Studies, University of Edinburgh. Lecturer in Psychology, Queen Margaret College, Edinburgh.
As a health visitor, Jenifer Holden became interested in postnatal depression. After studying psychology and counselling she helped to develop a means of identifying depressed mothers, who were then counselled by health visitors. This interest continues, and she also lectures in psychology.

Sally Inch SRN SCM
Practising (community) midwife in Oxford.
Sally Inch is the author of *Birthrights* and *Approaching Birth* (Green Print, 1989). She contributed to *Effective Care in Pregnancy and Childbirth* (OUP 1989) and has edited *Successful Breastfeeding – a Practical Guide for Midwives* for the Royal College of Midwives.

Marianne J G Mills RGN SCM
Community and Parenthood Department, Stobhill Maternity Unit, Glasgow.
Marianne Mills' initial research on teenage pregnancy began her interest in this subject. Previously she was Parenthood Sister at Stobhill and made a tape/slide programme on 'Breast for baby' with translated commentaries in Asian languages. She has also worked in New Zealand.

Rowan Nunnerley SRN SCM ADM MTD DMS
Director of Midwifery & Gynaecology Nursing Services, Camberwell Health Authority.
In her previous posts, Rowan Nunnerley managed antenatal and postnatal

wards and co-ordinated district parent education services. She is interested in assisting the setting up of national standards of care for midwifery (client and staff) to ensure a high quality of care.

Joyce Prince BA BSc PhD SRN SCM
Formerly Honorary Lecturer in Psychology, Institute of Obstetrics and Gynaecology, University of London.
Joyce Prince worked as a nurse and midwife before transferring to higher education to read social sciences. Until her recent retirement she was a Research Manager with the DHSS concerned mainly with nursing and midwifery research. She has published on health and social issues.

Janet Rush RN BScN MHSc
St Joseph's Hospital, Hamilton, Ontario.
Janet Rush is a Director of Nursing Practice, Maternal/Child Care. Her research interests include evaluation of clinical routines, services and programmes in obstetric care.

Ellena M Salariya RN RM
Ninewells Hospital, Dundee.
Ellena M Salariya is a Senior Midwife (Research) and part-time higher degree student. Her publications include studies on breastfeeding, smoking habits in pregnancy, mother-child relationships and umbilical cord care. She was awarded a Florence Nightingale scholarship in 1981 and has travelled widely in the USA and Canada observing maternal/infant interaction.

Jennifer Sleep SRN SCM MTD BA
Royal Berkshire Hospital, Reading.
Jennifer Sleep is co-ordinator of nursing and midwifery research within the West Berkshire Health Authority. She has conducted a series of clinical trials designed to evaluate aspects of midwifery care largely related to perineal management both during delivery and following childbirth.

Chris Whitby RGN RM
Neonatal Intensive Care Unit and Transitional Care Ward, The Rosie Maternity Hospital, Cambridge.
Chris Whitby is a senior midwife and a council member of the Neonatal Nurses Association. She is co-author, with the late Jean Boxall, of a teaching video on transitional care, 'Being together' and has contributed to the *Midwives Chronicle*.

Foreword

I was particularly pleased to be invited to write this foreword on postnatal care. Enabling women and their partners to embark in strength upon the adventure of parenthood makes a crucial contribution to the welfare of each individual family and to society as a whole.

Postnatal care was once described as the Cinderella of maternity care, and one of little interest to newly qualified midwives (Robinson, Golden & Bradley 1983). This presented a paradox; postnatal care in Great Britain consumes more than half of the midwifery resources, but was considered of little interest or challenge, mainly because we lacked sound theory or research on which to base our practice, or to assess its appropriateness and effectiveness. No wonder most consumer surveys complained consistently and bitterly of conflicting advice from midwives!

The increasing amount of midwifery research during the last decade has changed that situation, and much of that research has been skilfully distilled by the authors in this book to form an invaluable framework for practice.

Making the necessary changes in current practice will be a challenging process but one which I hope the midwifery profession can cheerfully face. In the first two chapters alone Sleep and Inch demolish much of current practice based upon cherished but untested theories! And yet, when we read their work, it all seems so logical and sensible and important. As Sleep points out, 'a woman cannot tenderly cuddle her baby whilst experiencing severe perineal pain!'

The unexpected perinatal death of a grandchild in 1988 showed me the difference that skilled, sensitive and loving care can make to such a bitter blow. Such patterns of care are explored by Prince and Adams.

In her chapter, Rush reminds us that in many countries without a community midwifery service, parents undertake all the care of the umbilical cord themselves. Whitby's chapter on transitional care shows this change increases the degree of contact between the newborn and his family; which Salariya shows is so beneficial and enjoyable ... and postnatal care should be about enhancing the joy and delight of a new baby in the family. It also releases skilled neonatal nurses for the care of low-weight and seriously ill babies.

This raises the issue of ensuring the proper use of resources, a matter which is increasingly important as we face the challenges of the restructured health service and the demand from the World Health Organisation that each member state must institute methods of Quality Assurance by the year 2000. Nunnerley's chapter on this subject is particularly well timed. Standards of care are not only about the way we provide care but also about the type, range, availability and appropriateness of that care. Any practice, however well meant, which is not effective or appropriate is neither efficient, cost-effective, nor acceptable.

Perhaps one standard we should immediately set is that of ensuring that the wealth of material in this book forms the basis of the care standards in every postnatal ward and community midwifery team.

Jean A. Ball
MSc, DipN.RM, RGN

Preface

There is no doubt that the theory underpinning midwifery practice cannot be carved in tablets of stone but must be dynamic and change as new information becomes available. Despite this, it is really only in the last 30 years that research has begun to have any impact on midwifery practice and even now relevant information is not always easily available to practitioners. The Midwives Information and Resource Service (MIDIRS) and the 'Research and the Midwife' conferences have made an outstanding contribution, but standard textbooks are often sparsely referenced and full length research papers are time consuming to read.

This three volume series is intended to help to fill the vacuum which exists between the current state of research and the literature readily available and accessible to practitioners. The series offers midwives and senior student midwives a broad-ranging survey and analysis of the research literature relating to the major areas of clinical practice. We hope that it will also prove stimulating to childbearing women, their families and others involved with the maternity care services. The books do not pretend to give the comprehensive coverage of a definitive textbook and indeed their strength derives from the in-depth treatment of a selection of topics. The topic areas were chosen with great care and authors were approached who have a particular research interest and expertise. On the basis of their critical appraisal of the literature the authors make recommendations for clinical practice, and thus the predominant feature of these books is the link made between research and key areas of practice.

The chapters have a common structure which is described below. It is hoped that this will be attractive to readers and assist those reviewing existing policies or wishing to study a topic in still greater depth. Some knowledge of basic research terminology will prove useful, but its lack should not discourage readers.

We owe a debt of gratitude to many people: most of all to our authors who have worked so painstakingly to produce their contributions and many of whom have helped us in numerous other ways; to Sarah Robinson for her early encouragement and to our publishers during the development of the series; and, not least, to all those practitioners and students who made valuable comments on draft material.

We hope that many practitioners will use the books to increase their knowledge, stimulate their interest in research and improve and extend their own practice of the art and science of midwifery.

JA
VL
SR

■ Common structure of chapters

In fulfilment of the aims of the series, each chapter follows a common structure:

1. The introduction offers a digest of the contents;

2. '*It is assumed that you are already aware of the following ...*' establishes the prerequisite knowledge and experience assumed of the reader;

3. The main body of the chapter reviews and analyses the most appropriate and important research literature currently available;

4. The '*Recommendations for clinical practice*' offer suggestions for sound clinical practice based on the author's interpretation of the literature;

5. The '*Practice check*' enables professionals to examine their own practice and the principles and policies influencing their work;

6. Bibliographic sources are covered under *References* (to research) and *Suggestions for further reading.*

■ Further reading on research

The titles listed below are suggested for those who wish to further their knowledge and understanding of research principles.

Cormack D F S (ed) 1984 The Research Process in Nursing. Blackwell Scientific Publications, Oxford
Hockey L 1985 Nursing Research – Mistakes and Misconceptions. Churchill Livingstone, Edinburgh
Tornquist E M 1986 From Proposal to Publication: An Informal Guide to Writing about Nursing Research. Addison Wesley, Reading (Massachusetts)

Chapter 1

Postnatal perineal care

Jennifer Sleep

Following delivery, the activity and excitement which accompany the moment of birth are often superseded by a time of quiet enchantment. For many parents, the experiences of labour are momentarily forgotten as they delight in the miracle of their newborn. These are precious moments for the new family, moments to be savoured and treasured. This is a time when the midwife should safeguard the couple's privacy, if only for a brief span, before reality and routine intervene.

The postnatal period is a time when each mother has to adjust to physical changes and new emotional demands. These two aspects are inextricably linked; a woman cannot tenderly cuddle her baby whilst experiencing severe perineal pain, neither can she feel herself to be an attractive, desirable partner if she is incontinent of urine. Whilst acknowledging the interdependence of physical and psychological factors, this chapter largely seeks to explore the physical problems commonly reported by new mothers by reflecting on current practices in perineal care.

■ It is assumed that you are already aware of the following:

- The physiology of wound healing;
- The anatomy of the pelvic floor;
- Which drugs are secreted in breast milk.

■ Perineal pain in the early postnatal period

Perineal pain in the early days following childbirth is one of the most common causes of maternal morbidity. There is evidence to suggest that 23 per

1

cent of women report some degree of discomfort 10 days following normal delivery (Sleep *et al* 1984); for those who need instrumental assistance this rate is as high as 66 per cent (Grant *et al* 1989). Perineal pain is a source of distress and discomfort which may severely jeopardise the woman's recovery and adversely affect the relationship with her partner for a considerable period of time. The problem, therefore, has consequences for tens of thousands of women every year in Britain alone.

During this ten day period, the midwife is the only health professional to be in daily contact with the mother either in hospital or at home. Mothers are therefore most likely to turn to their midwife for advice about the best way to alleviate this distressing problem. This leads to direct or indirect prescribing by midwives. Direct prescribing includes specific treatments such as bath additives or herbal preparations which are available through many retail outlets; indirect prescribing requires medical sanction for pharmaceutical products including some analgesics and electrical therapies but the request is often instigated by the midwife.

■ Oral analgesics

There is a confusing choice of pharmacologically active preparations which can be taken by mouth to relieve pain. Several factors need to be considered in selecting the most appropriate agent.

1. The severity of pain to be treated. It is useful to categorise pain as mild, moderate or severe (Wallenstein & Hood 1975) and limit the choice to preparations with sufficient analgesic potency to alleviate each type of pain. Postpartum perineal pain is usually mild or moderate when classified on this scale, although a small number of women report the experience as severe.

2. The extent to which the drug is secreted in breast milk and if so, whether this holds any potential danger for the baby.

3. The risks of maternal side-effects such as gastric upset or constipation.

4. The relative costs of the alternative preparations.

There is anecdotal evidence to suggest a wide variation in what midwives advise for perineal pain. In a recently conducted survey of 50 English maternity units (Sleep & Grant 1988), the first line management was usually oral analgesia (78 per cent). There was a clear consensus that paracetamol was the first line therapy for mild to moderate pain (96 per cent). This seems a sensible choice for nursing mothers as the drug is largely free of unwanted side-effects. (Drugs & Therapeutics Bulletin 1986). A stock is available in most maternity units and it can be bought over the counter at many shops. A useful alternative may be one of the nonsteroidal, anti-inflammatory agents such as ibuprofen (largely retailed under the brand name of Brufen); little is secreted in breast milk and this too may now be bought across the counter, marketed as Nurofen. The main disadvantage of this drug is its cost (50 × 200mg Brufen tablets could be bought for approximately £1.75 in 1989 while 50 × 200mg paracetamol tablets were nearer 50p in price at the same time). There was, however, no agreement about which oral analgesic should be given for more severe pain (see Table 1.1). The most popular

Table 1.1   Oral analgesics for perineal pain

	Consultant units n=36 (%)	GP units n=14 (%)	All units n=50 (%)
Mild/moderate pain			
paracetamol	35 (97)	13 (93)	48 (96)
More severe pain			
co-proxamol (Distalgesic)	7 (19)	2 (14)	9 (18)
− paracetamol 325mg + dextroproxyphene 32.5mg			
co-dydramol (Paramol)	5 (14)	1 (1)	6 (12)
− paracetamol 500mg + dihydrocodeine 10mg			
co-codaprin (Codis)	4 (11)	2 (14)	6 (12)
− aspirin 400mg + codeine phosphate 8mg			
co-codamol (Paracodol; Panadeine)	1 (3)	2 (14)	3 (6)
− paracetamol 500mg + codeine phosphate 8mg			
dihydrocodeine tartrate 30mg (DF 118)	2 (6)	0 (0)	2 (4)
papaveretum (Omnopon) + aspirin	2 (6)	0 (0)	2 (4)
mefanamic acid 250mg (Ponstan)	2 (6)	0 (0)	2 (4)
buprenorphine 0.2mg (Temgesic)	1 (3)	0 (0)	1 (2)
ibuprofen 200mg (Brufen)	1 (3)	0 (0)	1 (2)

choices were combinations of paracetamol or aspirin with another analgesic, most commonly a codeine derivative. Given its tendency to cause constipation, codeine does not seem the ideal choice in this circumstance especially when other effective alternatives are available. Dextropropoxephene, which in combination with paracetamol is marketed as Distalgesic, is free of this effect although it is less popular than it used to be because of the risk of dependence and overdose. These risks would appear minimal in relation to the efficacy of the preparation in relieving perineal pain especially when the more potent analgesic is likely to be required for a relatively short period of time. The combination of an opioid such as papaveretum (Omnopon) with aspirin may be particularly useful for more severe pain. Although concern is widely expressed regarding the potential risk in exposing the baby to aspirin via the mother's milk, the drug is secreted only in low concentrations (Briggs *et al* 1986) so it may be worth considering its occasional use as a means of improving maternal comfort.

■ Cleanliness and hygiene

Vulval swabbing and bathing are widely recommended both as prophylactive measures in reducing the risks of infection and for the relief of perineal discomfort.

Only one study published to date has compared vulval swabbing using antiseptic solution with 'jug douching' using tap water (Martin *et al* 1957). The infection rates and the incidence of wound breakdown were almost identical in the two groups suggesting that one policy was no more advantageous than the other. Neither of these practices is currently in common usage largely as a consequence of early mobilisation of mothers following childbirth thus affording them the dignity and privacy of a bath, shower or bidet.

In a recent study (Sleep & Grant 1988a) 93 per cent of women who were questioned on the tenth day following vaginal delivery reported that bathing had relieved their discomfort. This observation was uncontrolled, however, and there is no knowing whether a similar proportion of women would have gained relief if they had not bathed at all or had used showers rather than baths. This may be an important issue especially when many maternity units are supplied with bidets, and showers are increasingly fitted in modern units and many new homes. In addition, there appears to be little consensus in the advice given to mothers by midwives regarding the frequency of perineal cleaning although, for the most part, the mothers themselves are probably well able to decide their own schedule.

Only one randomised trial has reported a comparison between warm and cold sitz baths (Ramler & Roberts 1986). Cold sitz baths were more effective in relieving discomfort especially immediately following the birth. In practice, however, it is difficult to imagine that many women would willingly choose cold, rather than warm, water as a therapeutic soak. Indeed 119 of the 159 women approached to enter the trial refused to participate in this study; the main reason given was their reluctance to immerse themselves in cold water − an understandable response under the circumstances.

One of the oldest 'remedies' for perineal and other trauma is the addition of salt to the bath water. It is still very popular; as many as 33 per cent of women were adding salt to their bathwater ten days after normal delivery (Sleep *et al* 1984). Salt is believed to soothe discomfort and to speed the healing process, but its precise mode of action is unclear. Claims that it has antibacterial or antiseptic properties remain unsubstantiated

(Ayliffe *et al* 1975). There is little consensus as to the amount of salt to be used; recommended quantities range from a heaped tablespoon in a small bath (Marks & Ribeiro 1983) to 3lbs in three gallons of water (Houghton 1940). In the only published trial 1800 women were randomly allocated to one of three bathing policies (Sleep & Grant 1988a); 600 mothers were asked to add measured quantities of salt to the bathwater, 600 were asked to add a 25ml sachet of Savlon bath concentrate and the remaining group were asked not to add anything to their baths in the ten days following delivery.

Overall, 89 per cent of the women complied. There was little, if any, difference between the three groups in terms of perineal pain or relief afforded at either ten days or three months postpartum. The patterns of wound healing were also similar in the three groups. On the basis of these results there is no case for recommending the use of salt or Savlon bath additive as a means of reducing maternal discomfort following delivery. An additional factor to be taken into account is the cost of these preparations; 100 women using additives for 10 days would spend £320 on Savlon and about £8 on salt.

The use of hairdriers in the drying of the perineum after washing is another widely recommended practice. There is little consensus as to whether the hairdrier should blow hot or cold air. Some advocate its use with conviction, whilst other raise serious doubts about its usefulness, or indeed its harmlessness (Wheeler 1988). There is at least a theoretical possibility that the drying effect applied to the sensitive, moist skin of the perineum may have a harmful effect which may result in increased pain and possibly delayed healing. There is no evidence that this is the case: on the other hand there is no evidence that this practice is safe. This procedure is in need of urgent evaluation.

■ Local applications

Midwives possess an armoury of topical remedies used for the symptomatic relief of perineal pain. Many of these are recommended on a trial and error basis and are met with varying degrees of success; few have been subjected to formal evaluation.

Sleep and Grant (1988b) reported icepacks as the most commonly used local treatment (84 per cent of units). These were usually made from frozen water filled fingers of rubber gloves, occasionally a commercial cryopack was used. Ice packs do appear to give symptomatic relief by numbing the tissues but this effect usually lasts for a very short period of time and there is no clear evidence of any long term benefit. Indeed the accompanying vaso-constriction may delay wound healing. There are also concerns that, as solid icepacks are difficult to position accurately at an anatomical site such as the perineum (especially in postnatal women who are for the most part ambulant), 'ice burns' may occur as a result of contact with the skin and surrounding tissues. For these reasons it may be preferable to use crushed ice 'sandwiched' between layers of a pad which may then be applied for restricted periods of time when the mother is able to rest.

☐ Anaesthetics

These are currently available contained in a range of base carriers including aerosol sprays, gels, cream or foam. The agent of choice appears to be lignocaine. Three randomised trials have recently been reported assessing a variety of spray formulae each containing lignocaine. In the first of these (Harrison & Brennan 1987a), alcoholic aerosol formulations of 5 per cent lignocaine and 2 per cent cinchocaine were compared with water only placebo spray in a single dose study in 76 primiparae. Both anaesthetics were clearly more effective than water in relieving discomfort. Of the two active preparations lignocaine was marginally more efficient. In the second trial (Harrison & Brennan 1987b), lignocaine was used in both an aqueous and an alcoholic base; the aqueous preparation appeared slightly more effective than the alcoholic sprays containing either lignocaine or cinchocaine. The results of the third study confirm this finding (Harrison & Brennan 1987c). The analgesic effectiveness of 5 per cent aqueous lignocaine spray was superior to the alcoholic formulation and comparable to a single 500mg dose of mefanamic acid (Ponstan). The only reported side effect was transitory stinging following application of the alcoholic spray which may prove a deterrent to their repeated use by women following childbirth.

Lignocaine in a gel was compared to an aqueous cream (BNF) applied in the first 48 hours after delivery. The mothers who applied lignocaine reported less pain and better pain relief (Hutchins et al 1985).

There are claims that the repeated application of local anaesthetics in close proximity to mucous membranes can cause irritation and local sensitisation leading to discomfort. No evidence can be found to substantiate these claims. In the absence of such evidence it would seem that lignocaine, in an aqueous base, could prove a useful application for women in the relief of perineal discomfort. The gel formulation has the added advantage of being considerably cheaper – and ozone friendly. Prices for 1989 suggest that lignocaine spray would be 8 times more expensive than 2 per cent lignocaine gel containing 0.25 per cent chlorhexidine.

☐ Combinations of local anaesthetics and topical steroids

It is assumed that local oedema and inflammation are major contributory factors to perineal pain. In recent years pharmaceutical preparations have been developed and introduced into clinical care amidst enthusiastic claims for their efficacy in reducing these problems. Epifoam (Stafford Miller Ltd) is one such vigorously marketed product; it contains pramoxine hydrochloride 1 per cent and hydrocortisone acetate 1 per cent in a water-miscible muco-adhesive foam base. The only encouraging results on the use of this preparation have been from studies which were uncontrolled (Nenno *et al* 1973; Bouis *et al* 1981) or unsatisfactorily controlled (Goldstein *et al* 1977). In the only well controlled, double-blind study published to date (Greer & Cameron 1984) mothers in the Epifoam group reported more oedema and a greater use of oral analgesia, particularly after the third day, than mothers in the control group who used a simple aqueous foam. Wound breakdown was also more common in the actively treated group. In this study, outcome was assessed by an observer who did not know the trial allocation thus minimising assessor bias. Steroids are known to impair wound healing (Walter & Israel 1979) so it is biologically plausible that Epifoam may cause longer term problems in relation to perineal healing. Furthermore, it is costly (£3.00 per 12gm cannister was the approximate 1989 price), and Hutchins and his colleagues (1985) did not feel that the very marginal effectiveness over lignocaine suggested by their study warranted the extra expense. In the light of present evidence, it is questionable whether this product does have the benefits claimed for it; it should therefore not be recommended or prescribed for mothers until subjected to further longer term evaluation in properly controlled trials (Drugs and Therapeutic Bulletin 1987).

☐ **Herbal remedies**

An ever increasing number of herbal preparations aimed at relieving perineal discomfort is currently available through many retail outlets. Their growing popularity probably reflects a belief that 'natural' remedies must be safe. Some are produced in tablet form, others are recommended for infusion and external application. There is however a dearth of evidence to support their efficacy or safety (Ehudin-Pagano *et al* 1987).

Arnica (Leopard's Bane) is supplied as tablets; as it is claimed to stimulate tissue repair and to reduce bruising following childbirth a course of treatment is recommended to begin at the onset of labour or as soon after delivery as possible (Ford 1988). Chamomile and comfrey are both believed to aid healing; the latter may be steeped to form a solution which can then be mixed with slippery elm and applied to the perineum as a paste or added to bath water as a soothing soak (Bunce 1987). Swabbing of the perineum with tincture of calendula (Marigold) is also recommended because it is believed to have antiseptic properties, hence its advocated use also on the cord stump of the neonate. Rare cases of hypersensitivity to calendula have been reported (Drugs & Therapeutics Bulletin 1986).

In a recent survey (Sleep & Grant 1988b), 12 per cent of units reported the use of pads soaked in witch hazel as a locally applied compress. Two randomised trials have assessed this practice. Spellacy (1965) randomly allocated mothers to use either pads soaked in a witch hazel and glycerine solution or pads soaked in tap water. The majority of women in each group reported some symptomatic relief but there was no evidence that the witch hazel/glycerine combination proved any more effective in relieving perineal discomfort than plain tap water. The second trial (Moore & James 1989) was conducted in Bristol during 1986. Three hundred women who had forceps deliveries were randomly allocated to one of three treatment groups: witch hazel, icepacks and Epifoam. There was some evidence that witch hazel was the most effective analgesic on the first day of use, but by day three icepacks were the most satisfactory. Thereafter there were no clear differences between the treatment groups up to the final six weeks assessment.

Some herbal remedies may be potentially useful in helping mothers to recover after childbirth, however their widespread use needs to be approached with the same caution as the introduction of pharmaceutical products. Evidence is required that they are both safe and therapeutic.

☐ Electrical therapies

Ultrasound and, to a lesser extent, pulsed electromagnetic therapy are increasingly being used in the first few days after delivery to relieve perineal pain and discomfort. In a telephone survey of 36 consultant units and 14 GP units (Sleep & Grant 1988b), 36 per cent of units reported using ultrasound, 12 per cent used heat and 6 per cent used pulsed electromagnetic energy. These therapies were more frequently available at consultant rather than GP units.

The mechanisms by which therapeutic ultrasound may improve tissue repair and reduce pain have been reviewed by Dyson (1987). The precise mode of action is not properly understood but there is evidence that it is effective for some soft tissue injuries, such as tennis elbow (Binder et al 1985), leg ulcers (McDiarmid et al 1985; Callam et al 1987) and following oral surgery (El Hag et al 1985). Two small trials assessing its use for perineal trauma have been incompletely reported (McLaren 1984; Creates 1987). The transducer head is applied directly to the skin and must be moved gently throughout the transmission to minimise tissue damage by heating and air cavitation; conduction is aided by the use of a couplant jelly or cream. The therapy requires constant operator attendance and so is costly in physiotherapists' time.

Pulsed electromagnetic energy therapy is also claimed to improve wound healing and reduce pain. One of the greatest practical advantages of the treatment lies in its ease of application. It may be transmitted through a sanitary towel, so obviating the need for bedside attendance, although for safety's sake the physiotherapist needs to remain in the vicinity whilst any electrical treatment is in progress. One published study evaluating its use in perineal care suggests that active therapy accelerates the resolution of bruising (Bewley 1986). In this trial 100 mothers were randomly allocated to receive a treatment from one of two machines, one active and the other inactive. By day three of the trial, however, the author comments that it became obvious to the operators which was the 'active' machine. This may therefore have introduced observer bias on the part of the physiotherapists as well as influencing the mothers' expectations of the therapy. Perineal pain reported by the mothers before and after treatment failed to reveal any benefit from the active therapy.

A recently published study evaluated both these electrical therapies in a trial where each mode of treatment was compared in a 'double-blind' design (Grant *et al* 1989). Four hundred and fourteen women with moderate or severe perineal trauma were randomly allocated to receive active ultrasound, active pulsed electromagnetic energy, or corresponding placebo therapies. Operator, subject and assessor bias were minimised by using a twelve point dial on each machine: eight settings were active, four were inactive. The codes for the switches were held in sealed envelopes and changed at two monthly intervals to minimise the risk of participants breaking the operating code; the output of the machines was tested weekly by someone who worked in a different part of the hospital. Therapy was started within 24 hours of delivery, a maximum of three treatments being

Table 1.2 Ultrasound and pulsed electromagnetic therapies for perineal trauma: outcome 10 days after delivery

	Pulsed electromagnetic energy (n=129)		Ultrasound (n=134)		Placebo (n=131)	
	n	(%)	n	(%)	n	(%)
Perineal pain in last 24 hours*						
(reported by mother)						
None	33	(26)	53	(40)	48	(37)
Mild	57	(44)	50	(37)	44	(34)
Moderate	30	(23)	24	(18)	33	(25)
Severe	9	(7)	7	(5)	6	(5)
Use of pain-killers in previous 24 hrs	31	(24)	30	(22)	25	(19)
Community midwife's assessment						
Perineal wound breaking down	6	(5)	6	(4)	3	(2)
Haemorrhoids	33	(26)	35	(26)	33	(25)
Bruising	22	(17)	14	(10)	18	(14)
Oedema	13	(10)	10	(7)	11	(8)

* $P<0.05$

given during a 36 hour period. Mothers assessed their pain both before and after each treatment, at ten days and at three months postpartum. Overall, more than 90 per cent thought that treatment made their problem better. Bruising looked more extensive following ultrasound therapy but then seemed to resolve more quickly but mothers did not report less pain as a consequence. More pain was reported by mothers who had received pulsed electromagnetic energy therapy at ten days postpartum (see Table 1.2), although by three months following delivery there were no reported differences in outcome. Neither treatment had an effect on perineal oedema or haemorrhoids. In the light of these results current enthusiasm for these new therapies should be tempered. Further controlled trials are needed to replicate this design and to assess different machine settings and length of treatment.

■ Pelvic floor exercises

The main reason for teaching and encouraging women to perform pelvic floor muscle exercises is to prevent urinary stress incontinence and genital prolapse. It has been argued that pregnancy (Francis 1960) and childbirth (Kegel 1956) may be precipitating or aggravating factors for stress incontinence. Certainly the symptom is a source of considerable embarrassment and distress to women. The most marked difference is between nulliparous and parous women; 60 per cent of primiparae experience the symptom for the first time during pregnancy (Stanton et al 1980); for multiparae there seems to be relatively little increase in severity until parity reaches four or more (Thomas et al 1980). The problem usually resolves in the first few weeks postpartum but persists in an important minority. In a study of 1000 mothers following normal, vaginal deliveries, 19 per cent reported some degree of involuntary loss of urine three months post partum (Sleep et al 1984). Two contentious issues arise in relation to urinary incontinence and childbirth; perineal trauma at delivery as a precipitating/aggravating factor, and the role of pelvic floor exercises as both a preventative and a curative therapy.

There is a growing body of evidence to suggest that the risk of incontinence is not directly related to the extent of trauma to the perineal tissues at delivery (Yarnell et al 1982; Gordon & Logue 1985). A longer term follow up of 1000 women, conducted three years following normal deliveries (Sleep & Grant 1987) did not provide evidence to support the hypothesis that the liberal use of episiotomy prevents urinary incontinence (see Table 1.3). Several authors have recently suggested that faecal and urinary incontinence result from damage to the innervation of pelvic floor muscles, rather than stretching *per se* (Snooks et al 1984; Swash 1988). Whatever the underlying cause, weakness of the pelvic floor muscles, as

Table 1.3 Urinary incontinence three years after participation in a randomised
trial of restrictive versus liberal use of episiotomy

	Restrictive policy n=329 (%)	Liberal policy n=345 (%)
Involuntary loss of urine		
Less than once a week	69 (22)	82 (25)
1–2 times in last week	37 (12)	35 (11)
3 or more times in last week	6 (2)	7 (2)
Sufficiently severe to wear a pad		
– sometimes	26 (8)	24 (7)
– everyday	5 (2)	4 (1)
Loss of urine when coughing, laughing or sneezing	103 (33)	105 (31)
Loss of urine when urgent desire to pass urine but no toilet nearby	41 (13)	41 (13)

judged by an inability to contract them voluntarily and effectively, often
accompanies stress incontinence (Shepherd 1983). Exercises aimed at
increasing awareness and improving tone are therefore often recommended
and taught both during pregnancy and following childbirth. There is some
evidence that the more successfully the exercises are performed, the better
the results (Shepherd 1983). It is, however, difficult to know whether the
muscles are being contracted effectively without inserting a finger into the
vagina or the use of a teaching aid such as a perineometer gauge. The latter
consists of a rubber device resembling a foley catheter or a condom which
can be inserted into the vagina and inflated until the woman is just conscious of pressure. As the levator muscles are contracted, so the squeeze
pressure registers in cm water on the gauge thus enabling the woman to
know whether or not she is contracting the muscles effectively.

Neither of these strategies would seem to be appropriate for women in
the early weeks following delivery when the vagina and surrounding tissues
may be bruised and sore for some considerable time.

Few formal attempts have been made to evaluate the role of pelvic floor
exercises in this context. One such study, however, was conducted in 1985
(Sleep & Grant 1987). The aim of this study was to compare the postnatal
exercise programme currently in operation in the West Berkshire Health
District with a scheme which reinforced this initial instruction during the
immediate postpartum period. The reinforcement programme comprised
additional teaching sessions, positive encouragement by community midwives and health visitors, and attempts to enhance motivation by personal
contact and the use of an exercise diary for one month. The main hypothesis

was that the more intensive programme would reduce the incidence of urinary incontinence three months after delivery. Assessment also included the effect of the programme on perineal discomfort and the mothers' reported feelings of general well-being. One thousand, eight hundred women entered the trial and were randomly allocated to one of the two policies. By the time of the community midwife's visit on the tenth postnatal day, mothers in the intensive group were more likely to have performed their exercises than mothers allocated to the normal policy (78 per cent versus 68 per cent). This difference was greater three months after delivery (58 per cent versus 42 per cent). At three months postpartum, one in five women admitted some degree of urinary incontinence (5 per cent needing to wear a pad for some or all of the time), and 3 per cent had faecal incontinence. These frequencies were very similar in the 2 groups allocated different exercise policies. One of the differences observed was in the perineal pain reported three months following delivery. This was not, however, reflected in differences in dyspareunia or in the timing of resumption of sexual intercourse (see Table 1.4). The results of this study, therefore, do not support the primary hypothesis, and this in turn raises questions about the value and content of the exercise programmes currently offered to women around the time of childbirth. Gordon and Logue (1985) suggest that regular physical exercise which women find both interesting and fun (for example, swiming, dancing or keep fit programmes) might

Table 1.4   Perineal symptoms at three months postpartum

	Normal exercises n=793 (%)	Intensive exercises n=816 (%)
Pain in the past week**	101 (12.7)	76 (9.3)
– mild	69 (8.7)	60 (7.4)
– moderate	28 (3.5)	15 (1.8)
– severe	4 (0.5)	1 (0.1)
Time to resumption of sexual Intercourse		
– in first month	263 (33.2)	249 (30.5)
– in second month	351 (44.3)	380 (46.6)
– in third month	67 (8.4)	85 (10.4)
– too painful	13 (1.6)	9 (1.1)
– not attempted	90 (11.3)	85 (10.4)
– not recorded	9 (1.1)	8 (1.0)
Intercourse painful at first	368 (46.4)	391 (47.9)
Intercourse still painful	154 (19.4)	167 (20.5)

** X_2 (ldf) for trend = 7.14; $p < 0.01$

prove more therapeutic in the long term than encouraging them to practice specific pelvic floor exercises. It is possible that the substantial resources involved in teaching the current pre- and postpartum programmes could be used more effectively. Even a relatively small reduction in the incidence of this distressing condition is potentially important. Further well designed studies are therefore needed to assess alternative strategies aimed at prevention and treatment.

■ Recommendations for clinical practice in the light of currently available evidence

1. There is little evidence to support many of the midwifery practices or the advice mothers' receive relating to perineal care following childbirth. Overall, the quality of personal, individualised postpartum care is likely to be a major influence in reducing perineal pain and speeding recovery.

2. Paracetamol is the oral analgesic of choice for mild perineal pain. If this proves ineffective, a nonsteroidal anti-inflammatory agent such as ibuprofen may prove a useful alternative. For more severe pain drugs containing a codeine derivative should be avoided and combined agents such as oral papaveretum and aspirin considered.

3. Mothers appear to find bathing both therapeutic and desirable. If an ardent preference is expressed for the use of an additive such as salt, there is no evidence that this will prove harmful. As its addition does not appear to confer any specific benefit, however, its use need not be advocated.

4. The local application of ice should be approached with caution. Cooling with crushed ice should be considered for short periods only, preferably applied while the mother is resting. Tap water and witch hazel may be useful alternative cooling agents. The application of a local anaesthetic such as 5 per cent lignocaine spray or lignocaine gel are also effective in reducing discomfort and may last for longer. The addition of a steroid to such topical preparations should be avoided as this may impair healing considerably in the long term.

5. The use of herbal remedies should also be approached with caution. On the whole there is no good evidence that they are beneficial and some may prove to be harmful.

6. On the basis of evidence currently available personalised physiotherapy services such as therapeutic ultrasound, pulsed electromagnetic energy and the teaching of pelvic floor exercises may

prove beneficial largely as a consequence of the sympathetic, individualised support offered rather than the therapies themselves.

7. Overall what emerges is the need for midwives to give, and for mothers to receive, kindness, respect, understanding and patience. This is especially important in the early days following childbirth. Such a supportive environment should not be created as an 'optional extra available to some women because of their special needs ... but one which is an integral part of the organisational framework of the service' (Ball 1987). Such concepts of care then become 'woman centred', rather than routine or treatment centred, and may have a substantial impact in minimising pain and discomfort and promoting physical recovery and self confidence. This is the midwifery challenge.

■ Practice check

- What oral analgesics are most commonly prescribed for nursing mothers on your unit? What is the rationale for this choice? When was the policy last reviewed?

- In your health district have the midwives defined and documented standards of care relating to aspects of postnatal perineal management? If so, how much are these standards actually used in daily assessment – especially in relation to the measurement of the quality of midwifery care?

- Review the guidelines for practice/procedure manual currently available in your area of work. How rigid are they in their recommendations? What is the most recent review date given at the end of a document and how long ago is the oldest? Are references cited in support of the suggested actions? What practices would you like to question?

□ Acknowledgement

The author gratefully acknowledges the support of colleagues at the National Perinatal Epidemiology Unit, Oxford, in particular Dr Adrian Grant, Epidemiologist, without whose help much of this work would not have been undertaken.

■ References

Ayliffe G A B, Babb J R, Collins R J, Davies J, Deverill C, Varney J 1975
Disinfection of baths and bathwater. Nursing Times   71 (37) Supplement:
22–3

Ball J A 1987 Reactions to motherhood. Cambridge University Press, Cambridge

Bewley E L 1986 The megapulse trial at Bristol. Association of Chartered
Physiotherapists in Obstetrics and Gynaecology Journal   58: 16

Binder A, Hodge G, Greenwood A M, Hazleman B L, Page P, Thomas D P 1985
Is therapeutic ultrasound effective in treating soft tissue lesions? British
Medical Journal   290: 512–14

Bouis P J J, Martinez L A, Hambrick T L 1981 Epifoam (hydrocortisone acetate)
in the treatment of post episiotomy patients. Current Therapeutic Research
30: 912–16

Bunce K L 1987 The use of herbs in midwifery. Journal of Nurse–Midwifery
32: 255–59

Callam M J, Harper D R, Dale J J, Ruckley C V, Prescott R J 1987 A controlled
trial of weekly ultrasound therapy in chronic leg ulceration. Lancet   ii:
204–06

Creates V 1987 A study of ultrasound treatment to the painful perineum after
childbirth. Physiotherapy   73: 162–65

Drugs and Therapeutics Bulletin 1986 Herbal medicines – safe and effective?
24: 97–100

Drugs and Therapeutics Bulletin 1987 Epifoam after childbirth for perineal
pain.   25: 39–40

Dyson M 1987 Mechanisms involved in therapeutic ultrasound.
Physiotherapy   73: 116–20

Ehudin-Pagano E, Paluzzi P A, Ivory L C, McCartney M 1987 The use of herbs
in nurse-midwifery practice. Journal of Nurse–Midwifery   32: 260–62

El Hag M, Coghlan K, Christmas P, Harvey W, Harris M 1985 The
anti-inflammatory effects of dexamethazone and therapeutic ultrasound in
oral surgery. British Journal of Oral Maxillofacial Surgery   23: 17–23

Ford J 1988 Postnatal homeopathic treatment. Midwives Chronicle   101 (1206):
222–24

Francis W J A 1960 The onset of stress incontinence. Journal of Obstetrics and
Gynaecology of the British Commonwealth   67: 899–903

Gordon H, Logue M 1985 Perineal muscle function after childbirth. Lancet   ii:
123–35

Goldstein P J, Lipmann M, Leubehusen J 1977 A controlled trial of two local
agents in postepisiotomy pain and discomfort. Southern Medical Journal   70:
806–08

Grant A, Sleep J, McIntosh J, Ashurst H 1989 Ultrasound and pulsed
electromagnetic energy treatment for perineal trauma: a randomised
placebo-controlled trial. British Journal of Obstetrics and Gynaecology   96:
434–39

Greer I A, Cameron A D 1984 Topical pramoxine and hydrocortisone foam
versus placebo in relief of post partum episiotomy symptoms and wound
healing. Scottish Medical Journal   29: 104–06

Harrison R F, Brennan M 1987a Evaluation of two local anaesthetic sprays for the relief of post-episiotomy pain. Current Medical Research Opinion   10: 364–69

Harrison R F, Brennan M 1987b A comparison of alcoholic and aqueous formulations of local anaesthetic as a spray for the relief of post-episiotomy pain. Current Medical Research Opinion   10: 370–74

Harrison R F, Brennan M 1987c Comparisons of two formulation of lignocaine spray with mefanamic acid in the relief of post-episiotomy pain: a placebo-controlled study. Current Medical Research Opinion   10: 375–79

Houghton M 1940 Aids to practical nursing. Ballière Tindall & Cox, London

Hutchins C J, Ferreira C J, Norman-Taylor J Q 1985 A comparison of local agents in the relief of discomfort after episiotomy. Journal of Obstetrics and Gynaecology   6: 45–56

Kegel A H 1956 Early genital relaxation: new technique for diagnosis and non-surgical treatment. Obstetrics and Gynaecology   8: 545–50

Marks J, Ribeiro D 1983 Silicone foam dressings. Nursing Times   79 (19): 58–60

Martin R T, Reiss H E, Milne S E 1957 Vulval and perineal toilet in the puerperium. British Medical Journal   3: 670–73

McDiarmid T, Burns P N, Lewith G T, Machin D 1985 Ultrasound and the treatment of pressure sores. Physiotherapy   71: 66–70

McLaren J 1984 Randomised controlled trial of ultrasound therapy for the damaged perineum. Clinical Physics and Physiological Measurement   5: 40

Moore W, James D R 1989 A random trial of three topical analgesic agents in the treatment of episiotomy pain following instrumental delivery. Journal of Obstetrics and Gynaecology   10: 35–9

Nenno D J, Loehfelm G 1973 Clinical trial of a topical foam for episiotomies. Medical Times   101: 123–25

Ramler D, Roberts J 1986 A comparison of cold and warm sitz baths for relief of postpartum perineal pain. Journal of Obstetric, Gynaecologic and Neonatal Nursing   15: 471–74

Shepherd A M 1983 Management of urinary incontinence: prevention or cure? Physiotherapy   69: 109–10

Sleep J, Grant A, Garcia J, Elbourne D, Spencer J A D, Chalmers I 1984 West Berkshire perineal management trial. British Medical Journal   289: 587–90

Sleep J M, Grant A 1987 Pelvic floor exercises in post-natal care – the report of a randomised controlled trial to compare an intensive exercise regimen with the programme in current use. Midwifery   3: 158–64

Sleep J M, Grant A 1988a Routine addition of salt or savlon bath concentrate during bathing in the immediate post-partum period – a randomised controlled trial. Nursing Times   84 (21): 55–7

Sleep J, Grant A 1988b The relief of perineal pain following childbirth: a survey of midwifery practice. Midwifery 4: 118–22

Snooks S J, Setchell M, Swash M M, Henry M M 1984 Injury to innervation of pelvic floor musculature in childbirth. Lancet   ii: 546–50

Spellacy W 1965 A double blind control study of a medicated pad for relief of episiotomy pain. American Journal of Obstetrics and Gynaecology   92: 272

Stanton S L, Kerr-Wilson R, Grant Harris V 1980 The incidence of urological symptoms in normal pregnancy. British Journal of Obstetrics and Gynaecology   87: 897–900

Swash M 1988 Childbirth and incontinence. Midwifery   4: 13–8

Thomas M T, Plymat K R, Blanin J, Meade T W 1980 Prevalence of urinary
   incontinence. British Medical Journal   281: 1243–45
Wallenstein S L, Hood R W 1975 The clinical evaluation of analgesic
   effectiveness. In Ehrenpreis S, Neidl A (eds) Narcotic research: 127–45.
   Marcel Dekker, New York
Walter J B, Israel M 1979 General pathology (5th ed.): 104. Churchill
   Livingstone, Edinburgh
Wheeler K 1988 Perineal wound healing (a letter). Midwives Chronicle   101
   (1200): 14
Yarnell J W G, Voyle J G, Sweetnam P M, Milbank J, Richards C J, Stephenson
   T P 1982 Factors associated with urinary incontinence in women. Journal of
   Epidemiology and Community Health   36: 58–63

■ Suggested further reading

Briggs G G, Freeman R K, Yaffé S J 1986 Drugs in pregnancy and lactation.
   Williams & Wilkins, London
Grant A, Sleep J 1989 Relief of perineal pain and discomfort after childbirth. In
   Chalmers I, Enkin M, Kierse MJNC (eds) Effective care in pregnancy and
   childbirth: 1347–58/9. Oxford University Press, Oxford

Chapter 2

Postnatal care relating to breastfeeding

Sally Inch

Breastfeeding is a normal, physiological process, and a natural consequence of giving birth. In many communities it is still the only reliable means of ensuring the survival and healthy growth of a newborn baby. In all cultures however breastfeeding, like coition, is a learned activity; only the ability is innate. This is equally true for other primates, as became evident when they began to be bred in captivity (Morgan 1985). Successful breastfeeding therefore depends on the acquisition of the basic principles, accurate information and practice. It does not depend on luck, skin colour, antenatal breast preparation, breast size or, in most cases, nipple shape (see the Chapter by J. Alexander on 'Antenatal preparation of the breasts for breastfeeding' in the volume in this series on, *Antenatal Care*). It will be strongly influenced by the quality of the help and information given to the mother in the first two weeks after the birth of her baby.

In some cultures the skills and information a woman needs are acquired subliminally through almost daily observation of babies at the breast, and the social support she receives from other women after the birth of her own baby. In others, women depend almost entirely on the skill and knowledge of their professional attendants around the time of birth. As breastfeeding has declined however (particularly in Western societies) so too has professional expertise. At the same time breastmilk substitutes have been promoted so successfully that many mothers (and worse still, many professionals) have come to believe that it is of little importance whether a new mother breastfeeds or bottle feeds her baby.

Recently, such comfortable illusions have been shattered by the publication of two well researched books: *Breastfeeding Matters* (Minchin 1985) and *The Politics of Breastfeeding* (Palmer 1988). Health professionals who have read these cannot possibly doubt the importance of their role in the promotion and establishment of breastfeeding. In view of this, very little comfort can be derived (in the UK) from the HMSO report on infant feeding (Martin & White 1988); for even though the majority of new mothers begin breastfeeding their babies many switch to bottle feeding during the first two weeks, a time when midwifery care is still intensive. Only 26 per cent of babies are still fully breastfed at four months of age.

Much of the professional ignorance which has contributed to this state of affairs has arisen partly from a constant stream of misinformation, sanctified and perpetuated in print, and partly from a lack of research-based information with which to replace it. Such information is vital to midwives if they are to teach, and to mothers if they are to learn. As breastfeeding is a learned skill, simply repeating 'breast is best' is about as useful 'as knowing that potatoes are edible without ever learning how to cook them' (Palmer 1988).

One of the best ways in which to test the usefulness of clinical interventions (some would say the only reliable way) is by means of a randomised, controlled trial. In this way all possible variables, known and as yet unknown, which might in themselves affect the outcome measure, are equally (randomly) distributed between all of the comparison groups, and the difference in outcome between the groups can reasonably be attributed to the intervention. For this reason a Register of Controlled Trials in Perinatal Medicine has been established at the National Perinatal Epidemiology Unit in Oxford, with the support of the Maternal and Child Health Unit of the World Health Organisation, 'as part of its mandate to assist member states to evaluate and develop appropriate health technologies' (NPEU 1985). This register contains almost all the random controlled trials in the world literature, from 1940 onwards, as they relate to perinatal medicine. Of the 2–3000 or so trials listed, over 100 relate to breastfeeding; it is on the basis of these, together with other observational and non-randomised cohort studies, that this chapter will challenge much of the misinformation currently disseminated and practised by health professionals.

It will argue, for example, that women do not need to follow precise instructions concerning their diet, fluid intake, care of their breasts or the timing of feeds.

It will argue that babies do not benefit from the regulation of their time at the breast, that night feeds are not optional extras, that routine test-weighing is not a useful tool, that healthy term infants do not need additional fluids, that nipple soreness and breast engorgement are not inevitable and that there are no 'magic wand' treatments for these conditions should they arise.

■ It is assumed that you are already aware of the following:

- The anatomy of the breast;
- The changes that take place in the breast during pregnancy and in the first week after birth;

- The physiology of lactation;
- The role of the lactational hormones.

■ Critical appraisal of the research literature

From the moment of birth, a healthy mother and baby possess between them all that is necessary for successful breastfeeding.

Removing the baby from his mother, restricting feeding times, giving fluids, nipple preparations, test-weighing and so on, are deliberate acts; and the 'burden of proof' properly rests with those who wish to intervene. Unfortunately, however, a great many interventions have been introduced without any evidence as to their benefit, and much of the research has been conducted long after the interventions have been absorbed into common practice. Many, if not all, of them have subsequently been shown to be of no benefit, and are often positively harmful from the point of view of facilitating breastfeeding.

■ Postnatal care within the first few hours of birth

□ Crédes prophylaxis

Crédes prophylaxis is the instillation of drops of silver nitrate solution into the eyes of a newborn baby, in an effort to prevent the growth of the gonococcus which, if present, may cause permanent impairment of vision or blindness. At the time of its introduction in 1881, gonococcal ophthalmia was a major cause of childhood blindness, and there was no effective treatment for gonorrhoea once contracted. The use of prophylactic silver nitrate thus became mandatory in many countries of the world. However putting even a 1 per cent solution of silver nitrate into the eye causes immediate pain, irritation and usually redness and swelling, which may persist for several days. Since the introduction and widespread use of antibiotics, which are highly effective against gonorrhoea and do not cause the pain and irritation of silver nitrate, many countries (including the UK) have now abandoned its use. In 1980, the American Academy of Pediatrics approved the use of tetracycline or erythromycin as alternatives, but some States' laws still require the instillation of silver nitrate at birth – as do other countries including Sweden. The only randomised controlled trial of Crédes prophylaxis so far conducted (Kallings & Wahlberg 1982) was too small to demonstrate its effectiveness, but neither did it show any effect on the duration of breastfeeding. The use of silver nitrate is associated, however, with a loss of eye contact and a reduction in affectionate parental behaviour, and these may adversely affect the developing relationship (Korner 1974; Klaus *et al* 1975; de Chateau 1976; Butterfield 1981; Wahlberg *et al* 1982). For fuller discussion of this topic, see Inch (1984).

☐ **Timing of the first feed**

No research has demonstrated a 'critical period' during which the first feed must take place if subsequent breastfeeding is not to suffer, but very little observation has been made of the spontaneous breastfeeding behaviour of a woman with her newborn baby. Widstrom *et al* (1987) reported the behaviour of 10 babies born to women who had received no drugs in labour. Spontaneous sucking and rooting movements occurred after 15 minutes, hand-to-mouth movement after an average of 34 minutes and spontaneous suckling after an average of 55 minutes. If most babies show signs of being ready to feed within the first hour after birth, it would seem appropriate to respond by making help with feeding a more prominent feature of labour ward care. A woman who has just given birth is likely to attach great significance to the way in which her baby responds to her, and a successful first feed may have a positive effect on breastfeeding (de Chateau 1980).

Controversy still exists as to whether it is the early contact or the early feed which affects breastfeeding success. Many researchers have examined these effects in combination (Sousa *et al* 1974; Sosa *et al* 1976; de Chateau *et al* 1977; Thomson *et al* 1979; Woolridge *et al* 1985), and all have demonstrated a beneficial effect on breastfeeding. In a study conducted by Salariya *et al* (1978), contact between mothers and babies seems to have been similar in both control and experimental groups. One group fed within 10 minutes and thereafter two-hourly another fed within 10 minutes and thereafter four hourly. In the other two groups the first feed took place 4–6 hours after birth, and thereafter two-hourly, or four-hourly. Both the study itself and the 18 month follow-up suggested that babies who were fed early were likely to remain breastfed for longer. For a detailed description of how this first feed might be conducted (Houston 1985; see Minchin 1985).

■ **Postnatal care within two weeks of birth**

☐ **Feeding technique**

Breastmilk is produced by the glandular epithelial cells within the breast. The glandular tissue is arranged in lobes, rather like the segments of an orange. Each lobe is subdivided into smaller sections containing clusters of

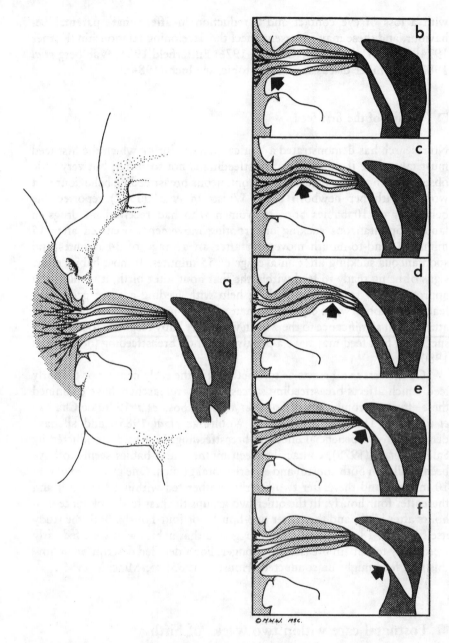

Figure 2.1 A complete suck cycle

sac-like spaces, or alveoli. Around each sac is a basket array of muscle (myoepithelial) cells, contraction of which enables the manufactured and stored milk to be released into the ductal system. Small ducts from each cluster of alveoli cells unite to form 10–15 larger ducts or lactiferous sinuses, which lie beneath the areola, from which milk can be removed. Using his tongue, the suckling infant exerts rhythmical cycles of compression to the teat formed from the breast and the nipple, squeezing milk from the ducts (see Fig. 2.1).

In order to obtain milk efficiently, both mother and baby must learn what effective attachment at the breast entails. The baby is equipped with reflexes that facilitate breastfeeding, but the mother (and the midwife) may be more familiar with the sight of a baby feeding from a bottle. Such familiarity often constitutes a considerable disadvantage, as the two processes have nothing in common, save milk transference. To begin with, a bottle fed baby has a bottle placed in his mouth, whereas a breastfed baby must be brought to the breast. The external appearance is also different, for a baby sucking a bottle teat uses the muscles of the face and jaw that an adult might use to suck a finger, whereas a baby feeding from the breast has his mouth open wide, using the muscles that an adult might use to suck a forearm. Neither are the bottle teat and the nipple in any way similar, for on the one hand the baby sucks on a rubber teat, centrally placed in his mouth, and on the other the baby feeds from a teat which is two-thirds breast tissue and one-third nipple. Also, the baby appears asymmetrically positioned at the breast, with more of the areola visible above the top lip than below the bottom one.

The bottle fed baby obtains milk by a combination of gravity and negative pressure applied to the teat; the process by which a baby removes milk from the breast is analogous to hand milking the teats of a cow's udder, whereby milk is expressed by a rhythmical, rolling action of the fingers against the teat in the palm of the hand. In the case of breastfeeding, it is the baby's tongue that performs this rolling action, as it works on the lactiferous (lacteal) sinuses within the areola. It is vital, therefore, that sufficient of the breast tissue is within the baby's mouth for the tongue to reach these sinuses. The nipple plays no active part in this process, and is simply the point of exit for the milk.

An appreciation of the qualitative difference between breast and bottle feeding is a necessary part of teaching good breastfeeding technique to the mother (see Figs 2.2 and 2.3). No attention should be paid to manufacturers who claim that 'their' teat is similar to the breast (Minchin 1985).

The precise 'anatomy of infant sucking' (Woolridge 1986a) is detailed in Fig. 2.1 above. This illustration shows how the nipple rests on the base of the tongue at the junction of the hard and soft palate and thus is not subject to friction from the gum. It should also be appreciated that there is no movement of the breast tissue in and out of the baby's mouth. The nipple is richly supplied with nerve endings and considerable pain results if it is

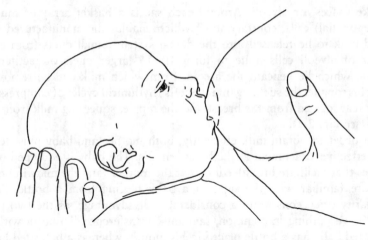

Figure 2.2 Poor breastfeeding technique: the baby is trying to 'bottle feed' at the breast

traumatised by the exposure to excessive 'negative pressure' (i.e. suction pressure – the way in which one draws liquid up a straw), pressure caused by the compression of the nipple between the tongue and the hard palate, or friction caused by the rubbing of the tongue against the nipple. All of these problems can arise if the nipple is not far enough back in the baby's mouth. If the baby is not stripping enough milk from the sinuses no milk flows and the initial suction pressure is maintained; meanwhile the action of the tongue is directed at the nipple instead of the breast tissue behind the nipple.

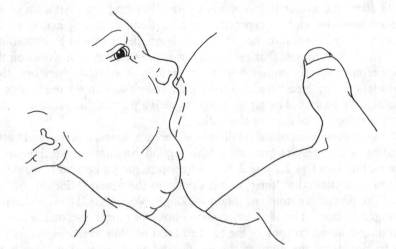

Figure 2.3 Good breastfeeding technique: the baby is well positioned at the breast

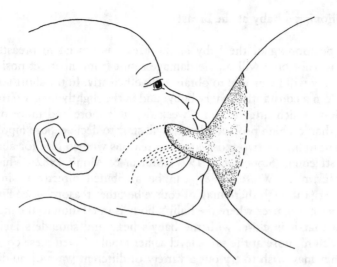

Figure 2.4 Poor positioning at the breast

Pain is a biological warning signal that damage is being done. In the context of breastfeeding, pain should alert the mother (and the midwife) to the fact that closer attention needs to be paid to positioning the baby at the breast (see Figs. 2.4 and 2.5). Pain should never be regarded as an inevitable consequence of breastfeeding for if it is ignored, severe nipple damage will result.

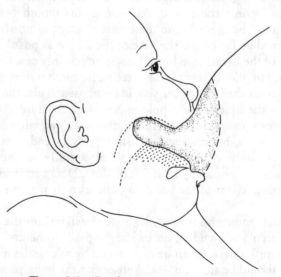

Figure 2.5 Good positioning at the breast

☐ Positioning a baby at the breast

Correct positioning of the baby at the breast is crucial to breastfeeding success, for not only will nipple damage result from incorrect positioning but the baby will be unable to obtain milk efficiently. In the short term this will result in a constantly hungry baby; and in the slightly longer term, milk production, which after the first week depends more and more on milk removal than on high prolactin levels, will start to decline. Sore nipples and insufficient milk, the two most common reasons women give for abandoning breastfeeding (Sloper *et al* 1977; Martin & Monk 1982; Whichelow 1982; Martin & White 1988), can be attributed directly to incorrect positioning (although there may of course be other reasons – see Fig. 2.6).

It does not matter where the baby's body is in relation to the mother's, provided that it is close, with the baby's head and shoulders facing her breast, with his nose at the same level as her nipple. Given these conditions the mother may wish to try out a variety of different ways of holding her baby. If the mother wishes to support her breast as the baby feeds, she should do so by cupping her breast in her hand, with her thumb on top and well away from her nipple. She should be strongly discouraged from using a 'scissor' grip, where the nipple protrudes from between the first and second fingers. This pushes the glandular tissue backwards, so that the baby cannot draw the lactiferous sinuses far enough into his mouth, and compounds the problem by having the lower finger where the baby's jaw needs to be.

The baby should be moved directly to the breast, with his head and body in alignment and his head slightly extended. It may be necessary, in order to elicit the 'gaping' component of the rooting reflex, to brush the baby's mouth against the nipple. As soon as his mouth begins to open widely, he should be moved onto the breast, gently but positively, and his lower jaw aimed as far below the base of the nipple as possible, so that he gets as much of the breast into his mouth as he possibly can. ('Below' in the above sentence implies that the baby is facing his mother directly; if he were lying across his mother's body she should be advised to aim the lower jaw as far *away* from the base of the nipple as possible.) Provided that the baby's shoulders are being supported, by the mother's, or midwife's hand, as he is moved to the breast, his head will remain slightly extended as he takes the breast. Thus not only will he be able to swallow easily but there will be no need to press the breast away from his nostrils. Doing so tends to pull the nipple upwards and out of the baby's mouth, as well as occluding the milk ducts.

An adequate mouthful from which to feed will include the nipple, some or all of the areola (depending on its size) and all of the underlying tissue including the milk ducts. It can be determined by asking the mother how it feels – there should be no pain – and observing the baby's sucking action. The jaw action should be rhythmical, and extend as far back as the ears, with no hollowing of the cheeks.

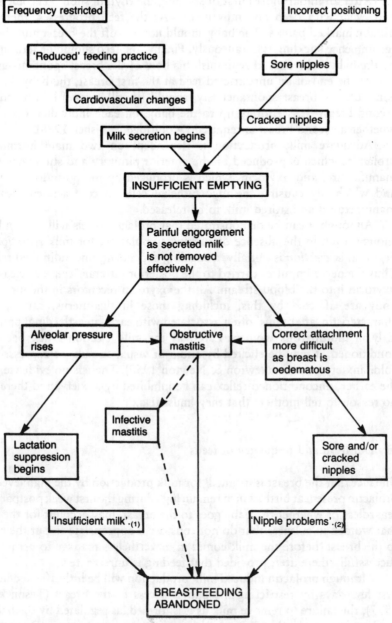

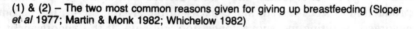

(1) & (2) – The two most common reasons given for giving up breastfeeding (Sloper *et al* 1977; Martin & Monk 1982; Whichelow 1982)

Figure 2.6 Possible consequences of a restrictive feeding schedule and insufficient early attention to the way in which the baby is attached to the breast

After an initial short burst of sucking, the rhythm should become slow and even, with deep jaw movements. As the feed progresses, there are usually marked pauses. The baby should not slip off the breast and should recommence suckling spontaneously. Finally, the feed should be terminated by the baby, who should relinquish his hold of the breast spontaneously.

At the end of an unrestricted feed at the first breast, the baby, having come off the breast spontaneously, should (if still awake) be offered the second breast. It is entirely up to the baby, on each individual occasion, whether a second breast is required (Woolridge & Fisher 1988).

Adequate milk production is dependent on two main hormones; prolactin, which is produced by the anterior pituitary and stimulates milk manufacture, and oxytocin, which is produced by the posterior pituitary and which, by causing the myoepithelial cells to contract, enables the manufactured and stored milk to be released.

Although it can be demonstrated that prolactin levels will remain high enough, even in the absence of sucking stimulation, for milk *secretion* to begin; milk *ejection* is initially, a suckling dependent, unconditioned reflex. Thus the nerve impulses carried to the posterior pituitary cause a release of oxytocin into the blood stream. All the oxytocin receptors in the mother's body are affected by this, including those in the uterus, causing the characteristic 'afterpains' often associated with early breastfeeding, particularly in multiparous women. Later, as the milk ejection reflex becomes conditioned, it may be elicited by audio or visual stimuli, or depressed by cold, anxiety or pain (Newton & Newton 1950). There is no evidence that the earlier, unconditioned reflex can be inhibited by anxiety, and therefore no reason to tell mothers that they 'must relax'.

☐ **Duration and frequency of feeds**

The fact that the breast is 'primed' for milk production by the high levels of prolactin present at birth, which remain high during the first week postpartum regardless of whether the baby goes to the breast, may account for the fact that women in cultures that do not consider it appropriate to put the baby to the breast 'before the milk comes in' nevertheless manage to breastfeed successfully thereafter, provided that feeding is unrestricted.

Although prolactin induced milk production will be little affected in the first few days by restricting the baby's access to the breast (Tyson *et al* 1977), the failure to remove milk as it is formed, as regulated by the baby's need to go to the breast, may have serious consequences. Once milk production exceeds the storage capacity of the alveoli, the breasts become engorged, resulting in venous congestion and pain. If this engorgement is sustained the back pressure on the milk producing cells results in the 'natural suppression' of milk production.

Milk production is a continuous process tailored to the needs of each individual baby. The younger the baby, the more likely he is to need the same volume of milk during the night as during the day (Dewey & Lonnerdal 1983). In physiological terms, the only reason for failing to remove milk from the breasts following childbirth is that the baby has died and the milk is not required. Just as importantly, from the standpoint of ultimate success of breastfeeding, unrestricted feeding from birth gives the mother and infant the opportunity to learn an efficient and effective feeding technique while the breasts are still soft, the baby still has nutritional reserves and the elevated prolactin levels are not yet wholly dependent on efficient suckling.

Each time the baby goes to the breast the anterior pituitary begins to release prolactin. Blood levels peak between 15–60 minutes later and have returned to basal levels within two hours of the feed. The prolactin response to suckling may be even greater at night than during the day (Hwang *et al* 1971; Glasier *et al* 1984). Although the basal levels and the amplitude of the prolactin response decrease over time (Glasier *et al* 1984; Howie 1985) this reaction to a feed can be demonstrated as late as 55 weeks postpartum (Madden *et al* 1978; Gross *et al* 1979), and sufficient milk to sustain healthy growth can be maintained for at least eight months (Ahn & Mclean 1980). It would seem that once lactation is well established, milk production is less dependent on high levels of prolactin, and more dependent on the efficient removal of milk from the alveolar sacs (Applebaum 1970). This in turn will depend on two major factors, the effective production of oxytocin in the mother, and efficient, effective milk removal by the infant.

Since the early part of this century, mothers have been (erroneously) advised to limit the time the baby spent at the breast. This damaging advice is still being offered to mothers (Stoppard 1982; Rice 1987) and to professionals (Ajayi 1980; Arneil & Stroud 1984) in the belief that it will prevent nipple damage. In 1981 Slaven and Harvey conducted a randomised controlled trial to test the effect of limiting sucking time. Not only did they fail to demonstrate any benefit in terms of nipple trauma, but significantly more of the women in the restrictive group had abandoned breastfeeding altogether by six weeks postpartum. These findings were supported by a study conducted by Carvahlo *et al* (1984). In view of the fact that healthy babies take very different lengths of time to take much the same volume of milk (Woolridge *et al* 1982), imposing restrictions on the time spent at the breast would, in many cases, decrease the volume of milk removed. This would in turn gradually decrease milk production. It would also, since the fat content rises as the feed progresses (Hytten 1954; Hall 1975), significantly curtail the calorie intake of many infants (Lucas *et al* 1979). It may also deprive infants of essential, fat soluble vitamins, such as vitamin K (von Kries *et al* 1987), and this practice may explain the increased incidence of haemorrhagic disease of the newborn in breastfed babies (Sutherland 1967).

The *frequency* of feeds has also, for ill-founded, historical reasons (Fisher 1982) been subjected to arbitrary limitations from birth onwards.

Observational studies, however, demonstrate that most infants feed infrequently in the first day or so after birth, but that the frequency rapidly increases between the 3rd and 7th day, and then decreases more slowly (Simsarian & McLendon 1942, 1945; Olmsted & Jackson 1950; Carvahlo *et al* 1982; Saint *et al* 1984; Carvahlo *et al* 1984). Furthermore, the interval between feeds, for the first few weeks at least, was found to be entirely random, ranging from 1–8 hours. Subsequently it has been demonstrated that babies who do not have feeding restrictions imposed, gain weight more quickly (Illingworth & Stone 1952; Salber 1956; Carvahlo *et al* 1983) and remain breastfed for longer (Illingworth & Stone 1952; Martin & Monk 1982) than those who do.

□ Supplementary fluids for infants

Despite the lack of evidence to support the routine use of supplementary water, dextrose or formula, this practise is still widespread (Garforth & Garcia 1989). The usual reasons given for this practice is that without additional fluids, babies may become jaundiced or dehydrated.

The volume of colostrum/milk produced by the breast increases rapidly, and the mean volume taken per feed increases from 7.5mls to 38mls in the first 48–72 hours. There is no evidence that a healthy term baby needs large volumes of fluid any earlier than they are available physiologically. Babies subjected to extremes of climate in Peru, Jamaica and the Middle East have been shown to maintain their urine osmolarity well within the normal range (Amroth 1978; Goldberg & Adams 1983; Brown *et al* 1986). The effects of giving water (Carvahlo *et al* 1981; Nicoll *et al* 1982) and dextrose (Kuhr & Paneth 1982; Nicoll *et al* 1982; Herrera 1984) to breastfed babies in order to reduce the incidence of jaundice, has also been studied; and found to be ineffective. One study (Kuhr & Paneth 1982) found that babies who took large volumes of dextrose were likely to take less milk from the breast, and another (Herrera 1984) found that babies who had received glucose supplements were significantly less likely to still be exclusively breastfed by three months of age. A further, randomised trial of formula supplementation (de Chateau *et al* 1977) demonstrated that the women whose babies were given formula were five times more likely to have abandoned breastfeeding altogether by the end of the first week, and twice as likely to have done so by the second week, compared with those whose babies received no supplements. This study has recently received further support (Gray-Donald *et al* 1985).

Those who give breastfeeding mothers free samples of formula to take home also reduce the chances that they will breastfeed successfully. Four random controlled trials (Bergevin *et al* 1983; Evans *et al* 1986; Feinstein *et al* 1986; Frank *et al* 1987) have shown that this policy reduces the likelihood that the baby will still be being breastfed 4–6 weeks later.

□ Supplementary fluids for mothers

The first study which demonstrated that increasing maternal fluid intake played no part in increasing lactation was conducted by Olsen in 1940. His findings have been supported by Illingworth & Kilpatrick (1953) and Dusdieker *et al* (1985). Additionally, Dearlove & Dearlove (1981) demonstrated that milk production is not affected by either significant increases or significant decreases in maternal fluid intake. Drinking large quantities of liquid, other than in response to thirst may be unpleasant and the accompanying increase in urine output may increase the discomfort to women with perineal or labial trauma.

□ Dietary modifications for mothers

Comparisons of the actual calorie intake of well nourished breastfeeding women with the recommended intake have consistently found it to be less (Whitehead *et al* 1981; Butte *et al* 1984). Furthermore, controlled trials of food supplements to undernourished women did not demonstrate an increased rate of growth in the infants of supplemented mothers (Blackwell *et al* 1973; Delgado *et al* 1982; Prentice *et al* 1983a; Prentice *et al* 1983b). Thus the nutritional demands of lactation appear to have been overestimated. Illingworth *et al* (1986) have subsequently demonstrated that metabolic efficiency is enhanced in lactating women, who are therefore able to meet the demands of their lactation even on as little as 1600–1800 calories per day.

Not only is there no evidence to support urging women to eat other than in response to their hunger, but there seems no reason, in general, to place restrictions on a woman's diet simply because she is breastfeeding. 'Allergic' disorders in breastfed babies, for which there is no other obvious cause, are often attributed to foods eaten by the mother (Gerrard 1980), but only the relationships between infantile colic and eczema appear to have been formally studied by means of randomised controlled trials. In the 20 colicky infants studied by Evans *et al* (1979) in a double-blind, cross-over trial, rates of colic in the infants were not found to be higher on the days when the mothers received cows' milk compared with the days on which they did not. In Jakobsson & Lindberg's study (1983), 66 infants with colic had cows' milk excluded from their (mother's) diet for one week, and then had it re-introduced. This challenge was done twice. Sixteen of the 23 infants who appeared to be sensitive to cows' milk then took part in a double-blind study which only 10 infants completed. Nine of these 10 reacted adversely to maternal ingestion of capsules of whey proteins, whilst none reacted adversely to placebo capsules. In a similar two phase trial, Cant *et al* (1986) examined the relationship between infantile eczema and maternal ingestion of eggs and cows milk. They found that only 6 of the 37 babies who entered the trial benefited from the exclusions.

It would appear that for both conditions there is a small sub-group for whom maternal dietary modifications may be helpful; and women with a family history of allergy may benefit from some modification of their diet, both in pregnancy and during lactation (Chandra et al 1986). A mother with no family history but whose child develops either eczema or colic, might reasonably be advised to try excluding eggs and cows' milk from her diet for two weeks and then re-introducing them. If the changes in the child's condition warrant permanent exclusion, the mother might need dietetic help to ensure her own nutritional adequacy. There seems to be no evidence for 'blanket' prohibitions of any foodstuffs for lactating women.

☐ Test weighing

The common rationale for routine test weighing of babies is to determine whether they have taken 'too much' or 'too little' from the breast. This presupposes that the weighing is accurate, that it is representative of the 24 hour intake, that professionals 'know' how much milk an individual baby should consume, and that action taken on the basis of the test weigh will do more good than harm.

The accuracy of the weighing will depend on who does the weighing; their accuracy; the accuracy of the scales and the degree to which the baby moves while being weighed.

The type of scale used for research purposes to collect normative data are heavily 'damped' integrated electronic balances. These produce readings accurate to within 2 gms, even if the baby moves vigorously, and a digital read out increases the accuracy of the recording. The type of scale most commonly found on postnatal wards are accurate only to within 10 gms, and this is further reduced if the baby is agitated. A study conducted by Stevens and Whitfield (1980; see also Whitfield et al 1981) compared the test weigh results of 96 bottle fed babies who had received a known volume of formula. The test weigh error was greater than 10 per cent in three quarters of the measurements, and exceeded 30 per cent in a quarter of them. Moreover the degree of error was most marked when the test volume was small; less than 60mls.

This poor correlation was also found by Culley et al (1979). In addition, Winberg and Wesser (1971) showed that, in a hospital where routinely test weighed breastfed babies were expected to take 10mls and 20mls respectively per feed on the first and second day of life, 98.5 per cent of them were deemed not to have done so.

There is some evidence that, if accurate electronic scales are used, there is a strong association between estimates of the volumes of single feeds and 24 hour intakes (Houston et al 1983), but an even stronger association between the volume of two feeds and the 24 hour volume. However it is also the case that feed volumes vary widely from feed to feed (Forsyth 1913;

Carvahlo *et al* 1982; Dewey & Lonnerdal 1983) and become less representative of the 24 hour volume after the first three days. Thus if it is necessary to know how much milk a baby is consuming, test weighing should be carried out at every feed for at least one 24 hour period, using electronic scales.

The energy requirements of individual babies are very difficult to determine, and are currently under review, as recent evidence (Whitehead & Paul 1981; Butte *et al* 1984; Wood *et al* 1988) suggests that the recommended averages may have been considerably over-estimated. Furthermore, the calorific value of breastmilk changes throughout a feed, and cannot easily be calculated (Hall 1975; Baum 1980; Saint *et al* 1984; Jackson *et al* 1987).

Finally, the only response to the results of the test weigh that will not do actual harm, is to pay greater attention to positioning the baby at the breast. The damage to lactation as a result of restricting feeds (if the baby has taken 'too much') or giving formula supplements (if the baby has taken 'too little') have already been discussed.

☐ **Prevention of nipple damage**

From the discussion (pages 23–26) of the 'aetiology of sore nipples' (Woolridge 1986b), it could be seen that incorrect positioning would be likely to lead to nipple damage. The most satisfactory way to prevent such damage is to ensure that the mother learns how to attach her baby to the breast effectively as soon as possible.

Attempting to keep the nipple clean, by the use of soap and water or alcohol in some form, has been shown to increase, rather than decrease, the incidence of soreness (Newton 1952). Commercial preparations in spray form, containing alcohol and chlorhexidine, have been shown to be ineffective in preventing nipple trauma (Slaven, Harvey & Craft 1976, unpublished, cited by Inch 1987; Herd & Feeney 1986; Inch & Fisher 1987). Of the creams and ointments that have been tested in controlled trials, the postnatal use of lanolin, silicone barrier cream, vitamin B ointment and vitamin A & D ointment have had no effect on the incidence of nipple damage (Newton 1952; Gans 1958; Shurtz & Kobermann 1978), neither has oral vitamin C (Gunther 1945). Stilboestrol cream and vitamin A & D concentrate have been shown to increase the incidence of damage (Newton 1952; Gans 1958). Tincture of benzoin, a commonly used preparation, contains 75–80 per cent alcohol and might, in view of Newton's findings, be expected to cause harm. Advising women to express colostrum or milk at the end of a feed and spread it over their nipple is no more effective than the use of lanolin in preventing damage (Hewat & Ellis 1987), but since the nipple is bathed in these substances throughout each feed it can clearly do no harm, and may be of psychological benefit to those who feel they must do something. Limiting sucking time, as discussed above, will not only be ineffective in preventing nipple trauma, but will also be deleterious to lactation.

☐ Treating sore nipples

The 1985 National Survey of Policy and Practice in Midwifery (Garcia *et al* 1987) elicited the fact that 32 different treatments for sore nipples were currently being offered to women in England and Wales. Of these, only three, re-positioning the baby at the breast, discontinuing feeding and expressing milk on the affected side and the use of a nipple shield have been evaluated by means of a randomised controlled trial (Nicholson 1985). During the 48 hour period during which these three treatments were compared, no statistically significant differences in nipple healing were detected, but use of the nipple shield was significantly less acceptable. Its use has also been shown (Woolridge *et al* 1980) to decrease milk transfer by 56 per cent in the case of the traditional shield and by 22 per cent in the case of the latex shield. 'Resting and expressing' for any length of time may also add to a mother's problems by gradually suppressing her lactation, as the prolactin response to the use of a pump is reduced, and less milk can be obtained from the breast (Friedman & Sachtleben 1961; Howie *et al* 1980; Howie *et al* 1985).

☐ Prevention and treatment of engorgement and mastitis

Because lactation is anticipated, the breasts are prepared anatomically and physiologically during the course of pregnancy (Smith 1974). Growth and proliferation of the alveoli and ductal system is stimulated by the increase in the levels of circulating oestrogen and progesterone, firstly from the corpus luteum and later from the placenta. Serum prolactin, under the primary control of the hypothalamus, also rises steadily from 8 weeks gestation until term (Sherwood 1971), but milk synthesis and secretion cannot begin until, following the expulsion of the placenta, circulating levels of progesterone and oestrogen have fallen to a point where they no longer inhibit the action of prolactin. Very rarely, retained placental fragments may prevent this decline (Neifert *et al* 1981).

The length of time between placental delivery and the beginning of active milk production varies, but seems to be on average 48–96 hours or 2–4 days post delivery. The supply of materials to the breast for milk production requires extensive cardiovascular changes in the mother. During this time there is increased blood flow to the breasts (as well as the gastrointestinal tract and liver) and an increase in cardiac output. Later, maintenance of these cardiovascular changes is suckling dependent (Lawrence

1985). At the same time as blood flow and cardiac output increase, milk secretion begins at the base of the alveolar cells where small droplets migrate to the cell membrane and are extruded into the alveolar ducts for storage (Kochenour 1980). Even if no suckling occurs, prolactin levels will remain high enough in the first week for a substantial proportion of women to start secreting milk (Neifert & Seacat 1985).

The degree to which women are discomforted by these early changes in the breast will probably depend to a large extent on how dramatically the blood flow to the breasts is increased – the so-called 'vascular engorgement'. Breast expression and the administration of oxytocics are of no value (Ingelman-Sundberg 1958) as the breasts are not, at this stage, overfull with milk (Ingelman-Sundberg 1958; Koshiishi *et al* 1971). Since the changes in blood flow and the start of milk synthesis are both a consequence of the uninhibited action of prolactin, however, it would not be surprising if there was a degree of overlap. Milk engorgement, on the other hand, is almost always iatrogenic due to the inefficient emptying of the breast as a result of incorrect positioning or the restriction of feeds (see pages 26–29 above).

Treatment should therefore be directed at the cause. Only if the engorgement has progressed to the point of inflammation and the flu-like symptoms of mastitis (Gunther 1973) should gentle expression of the breast, by hand or by pump, be attempted (Thomsen *et al* 1984).

Unresolved non-infective mastitis may progress to infective mastitis, for which antibiotics will be required. It need not be assumed that all instances of mastitis are caused by infection (Marshall *et al* 1975; Neibyl *et al* 1978) and recent evidence suggests that a differential diagnosis can be made rapidly on the basis of leucocyte and bacterial counts (Thomsen *et al* 1984) without waiting for the results of bacterial cultures.

Not uncommonly, women with mastitis are advised to stop breastfeeding. Marshall *et al* (1975) offered evidence that the chances of developing a breast abscess are increased, rather than decreased, by this advice. If the mastitis is due to bacterial infection, milk from the affected breast can be expressed and discarded until the condition has resolved.

■ **Recommendations for clinical practice in the light of currently available evidence**

1. All midwifery care should be research-based; midwives should pass onto breastfeeding women only those practices which have been demonstrated to be effective. They should be prepared and able to justify all of the advice that they give, both to mothers and to any one else they are called upon to teach.

2. A clear understanding of the mechanism of lactation, and the way in which a baby feeds from the breast is an essential prerequisite of

helping breastfeeding women. Expertise in helping women position their babies at the breast can only come with practice. Midwives should take every opportunity to learn from their more experienced colleagues, and from the mothers themselves.

3. No baby should be removed from its mother at birth without good reason, and the midwife who delivers the baby should expect to supervise the baby's first feed. If this is impossible, because the baby or mother need medical attention which precludes it, the mother should be reassured that there is no evidence that the timing of the first feed is, in itself, crucial to success.

4. No limitations should be placed on either the duration or the frequency of the breastfeeds of healthy newborns. Mothers should not be encouraged to record the length of the feed.

5. All breastfeeding mothers need to sleep within earshot of their babies, if not closer, and their babies should have the same unrestricted access to the breast at night as they have during the day.

6. Mothers should be advised to allow the baby to finish the first breast first; allowing the baby to come off spontaneously, before offering the second. It is then immaterial whether a baby takes both breasts or just one, at any particular feed.

7. Additional fluids for the baby, such as water, dextrose or formula, should neither be offered nor recommended to the breastfeeding mothers of healthy babies. No free samples of formula should be given to mothers either in hospital or on discharge.

8. Breastfeeding women should not be advised to increase their fluid intake beyond the dictates of thirst, nor to modify their diet in the absence of specific indications.

9. No healthy, term, breastfed baby should be routinely test weighed. Should it be necessary to know the actual volume of milk a baby is receiving, the weighing should be carried out over a 24 hour period, using a heavily damped electronic balance.

10. Mothers should be advised that breastfeeding should be a pain-free activity. If pain is experienced it should be regarded as a signal that feeding technique may need to be improved and the fact reported to their midwife.

11. Mothers should be advised that no cream, spray or ointment has yet been shown to either prevent or cure nipple damage; and no midwife should recommend them.

12. Provided that a mother with mastitis can be closely supervised, and the affected breast efficiently 'milked' either by the baby alone or in

conjunction with a breast pump, immediate recourse to prophylactic antibiotics (with their potential side-effects) need not be made.

13. No mother should be advised to wean her baby abruptly, particularly if her breasts are engorged or inflamed. The abrupt cessation of milk removal results in acute engorgement which may lead to mastitis and possibly abscess formation.

■ Practice check

● How would you respond to a mother who requested water for her breastfed baby? How would you justify your response?

● How would you advise a mother who complained of engorged breasts? What explanation would you give her as to the probable cause of her condition?

● How would you explain to a mother how long a breastfeed should last?

● What advice could you give to a mother who complained of sore nipples?

● How would you respond to a colleague on a postnatal ward who proposed to remove a (breastfed) baby from its newly delivered mother overnight so that the mother could sleep?

● What would you say to a breastfeeding mother who asked if she should buy some bottles and teats to keep at home 'just in case'?

● How would you reassure a breastfeeding mother who was anxious that the baby would not be able to breathe easily whilst feeding because he was so close to the breast when correctly positioned? Or that she would not be able to relax while feeding?

● How would you know that a baby was correctly positioned at the breast?

□ Acknowledgements

The author wishes to thank the following for their kind permission to use the illustrations that appear in this chapter:

Fig. 2.1. Dr M W Woolridge and the publishers Churchill Livingstone. This diagram first appeared in 1986, in Midwifery 2: 164–76.
Figs. 2.2, 2.3, 2.4 and 2.5. Royal College of Midwives. These diagrams first

appeared in their handbook *Successful Breastfeeding – A Practical Guide for Midwives*.

Fig. 2.6   Oxford University Press. This diagram first appeared in Inch S, Renfrew M J 1989 Common breastfeeding problems: chapter 81 of Chalmers I, Enkin M, Kierse M (eds) *Effective Care in Pregnancy and Childbirth*.

■ References

Ahn C H, McLean W C 1980 Growth of the exclusively breastfed infant. American Journal of Clinical Nutrition   33: 182–92

Ajayi V 1980 The normal infant. In Textbook of Midwifery: 145. Macmillan, London

Amroth S G 1978 Water requirements of breastfed infants in a hot climate. American Journal of Clinical Nutrition   31: 1154–57

Applebaum R M 1970 The modern management of successful breastfeeding. Pediatric Clinics of North America   17: 203–55

Arneil G, Stroud C 1984 Infant feeding. In Forfar J O, Arneil G (eds) Texbook of Paediatrics, 3rd edn, Volume 1: 259–77. Churchill Livingstone, Edinburgh

Baum J D 1980 Flow and composition of suckled breastmilk. In Freier S, Edelman A I (eds) Human milk, its biological and social value. Proceedings of the International Symposium on Breastfeeding, Tel Aviv, Israel. Excerpta Medica, Amsterdam

Bergevin Y, Dougherty C, Kramer M S 1983 Do infant formula samples shorten the duration of breastfeeding? Lancet   i: 1148–51

Blackwell R, Chow B F, Chinn K S K, Blackwell B N 1973 Prospective maternal nutrition study in Taiwan; rationale, study design, feasibility and preliminary findings. Nutrition Reports International   7: 517–32

Brown K H, Creed de Kanashiro H, Aguila R, Lopez de Romana G, Black R 1986 Milk consumption and hydration status of exclusively breastfed infants in a warm climate. Paediatrics   108: 677–80

Butte N F, Garza C, O'Brian Smith E, Nichols B L 1984 Human milk intake and growth in exclusively breast-fed infants. Journal of Pediatrics   104: 187–95

Butterfield P M 1981 Does the early application of silver nitrate impair maternal attachment? Paediatrics   67 (5): 737–38

Cant A J, Bailes J A, Marsden R A, Hewitt D 1986 Effect of maternal dietary exclusion on breastfed infants with eczema: two controlled studies. British Medical Journal   293: 231–33

Carvahlo M, Hall M, Harvey D 1981 Effects of water supplementation on physiological jaundice in breastfed babies. Archives of Diseases in Childhood   56: 568–69

Carvahlo M, Robertson S, Merkatz R, Klaus M 1982 Milk intake and frequency of feeding in breast-fed infants. Early Human Development   7: 155–63

Carvahlo M, Robertson S, Friedman A, Klaus M 1983 Effect of frequent breastfeeding on early milk production and infant weight gain. Pediatrics 72: 307–11

Carvahlo M, Robertson S, Klaus M 1984 Does the duration and frequency of early breastfeeding affect nipple pain? Birth   11 (2): 81–4

Chandra R K, Puri S, Suraika C *et al* 1986 Influence of maternal food avoidance during pregnancy and lactation on the incidence of atopic eczema in infants. Clinical Allergy 16: 562–69

de Chateau P 1976 Neonatal care routines: influences on maternal and infant behaviour and on breastfeeding. Medical dissertation, new series No 28. University of Umea

de Chateau P 1980 The first hour after delivery: its impact on synchrony of parent-infant relationship. Paediatrician 9: 151–68

de Chateau P, Holmberg H, Jakobsson K, Winberg J 1977 A study of factors promoting and inhibiting lactation. Developmental Medicine and Childhood Neurology 19: 575–84

Culley P, Milan P, Roginski C, Waterhouse J, Wood B 1979 Are breastfed babies still getting a raw deal in hospital? British Medical Journal 2: 889–91

Dearlove J C, Dearlove B M 1981 Prolactin, fluid balance and lactation. British Journal of Obstetrics and Gynaecology 88: 652–54

Delgado H L, Marmtorell R, Klein R E 1982 Nutrition, lactation and birth interval components in Rural Guatamala. American Journal of Clinical Nutrution 35: 1468–76

Dewey K G, Lonnerdal B 1983 Breastmilk intake: variations in breastfeeding practices. American Journal of Clinical Nutrition 38: 152–53

DHSS 1988 Report on Health and Social Subjects No 32. Present day practice in infant feeding. HMSO, London

Dusdieker L B, Booth B M, Stumbo P J, Eichenberger J M 1985 Effects of supplemental fluids on human milk production. Journal of Pediatrics 105: 207–11

Evans C J, Lyons N B, Killien M G 1986 The effect of infant formula samples on breastfeeding practises. Journal of Obstetric, Gynecologic and Neonatal Nursing 15: 401–05

Evans R W, Fergusson D M, Allardyce R A, Taylor B 1979 Maternal diet and infantile colic in breastfed infants. Lancet i: 1340–42

Feinstein J M, Berkelhamer J E, Gruszka M E, Wong C A, Carey A E 1986 Factors related to early termination of breastfeeding in an urban population. Pediatrics 78: 210–15

Frank D A, Wintz S J, Sorenson J R, Heeren T 1987 Commercial discharge packs and breastfeeding counselling: effects on infant feeding practises in a randomized trial. Pediatrics 80: 845–54

Fisher C 1982 Mythology in midwifery – or making breastfeeding scientific and exact. Oxford Medical School Gazette 33 (2): 30–3

Forsyth D 1913 Breastfeeding: the consumption of breastmilk. Lancet, June 14th: 1656–57

Friedman E A, Sachtleben M R 1961 Oxytocin in lactation. American Journal of Obstetrics and Gynecology 82: 846–55

Gans B 1958 Breast and nipple pain in early stages of lactation. British Medical Journal 4: 830–34

Gerrard J W 1980 Adverse reactions to foods in breast-fed babies. In Freier S Eidelman A I (eds) Human milk – its biological and social value. Selected papers from the international symposium on breastfeeding, Tel Aviv, February 1980. Excerpta Medica, Oxford

Garcia J, Garforth S, Ayers S 1987 The policy and practice of midwifery study: introduction and methods. Midwifery   3: 2–9

Garforth S, Garcia J 1989 Breastfeeding policies in practice – no wonder they get confused. Midwifery   5: 75–83

Glasier A S, McNeilly, A S, Howie P W 1984 The prolactin response to suckling. Clinical Endocrinology   21: 109–16

Goldberg N M, Adams E 1983 Supplementary water for breastfed babies in a hot dry climate – not really a necessity. Archives of Disease in Childhood   58: 73–4

Gray-Donald K, Kramer M S, Munday S, Leduc D G 1985 Effect of formula supplementation in the hospital on the duration of breastfeeding: a controlled clinical trial. Paediatrics   75: 514–18

Gross B A, Eastman C J, Bowen K M, McElduff A P 1979 Integrated concentrations of prolactin in breastfeeding mothers. Australia and New Zealand Journal of Obstetrics and Gynaecology   19: 150–53

Gunther M 1945 Sore nipples: causes and prevention. Lancet   ii: 590–93

Gunther M 1973 Infant feeding: 107. Penguin Books, Harmondsworth

Hall B 1975 Changing composition of milk and the early development of an appetite control. Lancet   ii: 779–81

Herd B, Feeney J G 1986 Two aerosol sprays in nipple trauma. The Practitioner   230: 31–8. (See also Inch & Fisher 1987, below)

Herrera A J 1984 Supplemented versus unsupplemented breastfeeding. Perinatology–Neonatology   8: 70–1

Hewat R J, Ellis D J 1987 A comparison of the effectiveness of two methods of nipple care. Birth   14 (1): 41–5

Houston M J, Howie P W, McNeilly A S 1983 Factors affecting the duration of breastfeeding: 1. Measurement of breast milk intake in the first week of life. Early Human Development   8: 49–54

Howie P W 1985 Breastfeeding: a new understanding. Midwives Chronicle   98 (1170): 184–92

Howie P W, McNeilley A S, McArdle T, Smart L, Houston M J 1980 The relationship between suckling induced prolactin response and lactogenesis. Journal of Clinical Endocrinology and Metabolism   50: 670–73

Hwang P, Guyda H, Friesen H 1971 A radio immunoassay for human prolactin. Proceedings of the National Academy of Science in the USA   60: 1902–06

Hytten F 1954 Clinical studies in lactation: 11 Variation in the major constituents during a feed.   British Medical Journal   1: 176–79

Illingworth P J, Jong R T, Howie P W, Leslie P, Isles T E 1986 Diminution in energy expenditure during lactation. British Medical Journal   292: 437–41

Illingworth R S, Stone D G 1952 Self-demand feeding in a maternity unit. Lancet   i: 683–87

Illingworth R S, Kilpatrick B 1953 Lactation and fluid intake. Lancet   ii: 1175–77

Inch S 1984 Birthrights. Random House, New York

Inch S 1987 Difficulties with breastfeeding – midwives in disarray? Journal of the Royal Society of Medicine   80: 53–58

Inch S, Fisher C 1987 Antiseptic sprays and nipple trauma. The Practitioner   230: 1037–38

Ingelman-Sundberg A 1958 Early puerperal breast engorgement. Acta Paediatrica Scandinavica   32: 399–402

Jackson D A, Woolridge M W, Imong S N *et al* 1987 The automatic sampling shield: a device for obtaining suckled milk samples. Early Human Development 15: 295–306

Jakobsson I, Lindberg T 1983 Cows milk proteins cause infantile colic in breastfed infants: a double-blind crossover study. Pediatrics 71 (2): 168–271

Kallings M, Wahlberg V 1982 Antibacterial effects of silver nitrate used for Crédes prophylaxis and of a colloidal silver compound – hexarginum. Acta Paediatrica Scandinavica 295 (Supplement): 37–42

Klaus M H, Trause M A, Kennell J H 1975 Does maternal behaviour after delivery show a characteristic pattern? In Potter E, O'Connor M (eds) Ciba Foundation Symposium 23 (new series). Elsevier, Amsterdam

Korner A F 1974 The effect of the infant's state or level of arousal, sex and ontogenetic stage on its caregiver. In Lewis M, Rosenblum L A (eds) The effect of the infant on its care giver: 105–21. John Wiley, London

Kochenour N K 1980 Lactation suppression. Clinical Obstetrics and Gynecology 23: 1052–59

Koshiishi T, Furusawa Y, Iseki H, Iwasaki Y 1971 A double-blind study of the effects of Kimotab on engorgement of the breast. Acta Obstetrica et Gynecologica Japonica 18: 222–28

Kuhr M, Paneth N 1982 Feeding practices and neonatal jaundice. Journal of Paediatric Gastroenterology and Nutrition 1: 485–88

Lawrence R 1985 Breastfeeding – a guide for the medical profession, 2nd ed. C V Mosby, St Louis

Lucas A, Lucas P J, Baum J D 1979 Patterns of milk flow in breastfed babies. Lancet ii: 57–9

Madden J D, Boyar R M, MacDonald P C, Porter J C 1978 Analysis of secretory patterns of prolactin and gonadotrophin during 24 hours in a lactating woman before and after resumption of the menses. American Journal of Obstetrics and Gynecology 132: 430–41

Marshall B R, Hepper J K, Zirbel C C 1975 Sporadic puerperal mastitis: an infection that need not interrupt lactation. Journal of the American Medical Association 233: 1377–79

Martin J, Monk J 1982 Infant feeding 1980. HMSO, London

Martin J, White A 1988 Infant feeding 1985. HMSO, London

Minchin M 1985 Breastfeeding matters. Alma Publications, Australia; Allen and Unwin, London

Morgan E 1985 The descent of woman, 2nd edn: 100; 223. Souvenir Press, London

National Perinatal Epidemiology Unit 1985 A classified bibliography of controlled trials in perinatal medicine 1940–1984. Oxford University Press, Oxford

Neibyl J R, Spence M R, Parmley T H 1978 Sporadic (non-epidemic) puerperal mastitis. Journal of Reproductive Medicine 20: 97–100

Neifert M R, McDonough S, Neville M 1981 Failure of lactogenesis associated with placental retention. American Journal of Obstetrics and Gynecology 140: 477–78

Neifert M R, Seacat J M 1985 Contemporary breastfeeding management. Clinical Perinatology 12: 319–42

Newton N 1952 Nipple pain and nipple damage. Journal of Paediatrics 41: 411–23

Newton N R, Newton M 1950 Relation of the letdown reflex to the ability to breastfeed. Paediatrics 5: 726–33

Nicholson W 1985 Cracked nipples in breastfeeding mothers: a randomised trial of three methods of management. Nursing mothers of Australia Newsletter 21: 7–10

Nicholl A, Ginsburg R, Tripp J H 1982 Supplementary feeding and jaundice in newborns. Acta Paediatrica Scandinavica 72: 759–61

Olmstead R W, Jackson E B 1950 Self demand feeding in the first week of life. Pediatrics 6: 396–401

Olsen A 1940 Nursing under conditions of thirst or excessive ingestion of fluids. Acta Obstetrica et Gynecolica Scandinavica 20: 313–43

Palmer G 1988 The politics of breastfeeding. Pandora Press, Allen & Unwin, London

Prentice A M, Whitehead R G, Roberts S B 1983a Dietary supplementation of lactating Gambian women 1. Effect on breastmilk volume and quantity. Human Nutrition and Clinical Nutrition 37 (c): 53–64

Prentice A M, Lunn P G, Watkinson M, Whitehead R G 1983b Dietary supplementation of lactating Gambian women II. Effect on maternal health, nutritional status and biochemistry. Human Nutrition and Clinical Nutrition 37 (c): 65–74

Rice I 1987 Breastfeeding: a heartstart. Dell books, New York

Saint L, Smith M, Hartmann P E 1984 The yield and nutrient content of colostrum and milk of women giving birth to one month postpartum. British Journal of Nutrition 52: 87–95

Salariya E M, Easton P M, Cater J I 1978 Duration of breastfeeding after early initiation and frequent feeding. Lancet ii: 1141–43

Salber E J 1956 The effect of different feeding schedules on the growth of Bantu babies in the first week of life. Journal of Tropical Paediatrics (September): 97–102

Sherwood L M 1971 Human prolactin. New England Journal of Medicine 294: 774

Shurtz A R, Kobermann M 1978 Comparison of nipple care in the puerperium with powder and ointment. Geburtshilfe Frauenheilkd 38: 573–76

Simsarian F P, McLendon P A 1942 Feeding behaviour of an infant during the first twelve weeks of life on a self demand schedule. Journal of Pediatrics 20: 93–103

Simsarian F P, McLendon P A 1945 Further records of the self demand schedule. Journal of Pediatrics 27: 109–14

Slaven S, Harvey D 1981 Unlimited sucking time improves breastfeeding. Lancet i: 392–93

Sloper K, Elsden E, Baum J D 1977 Increasing breastfeeding in a community. Archives of Disease in Childhood 52: 700–02

Smith V R 1974 The mammary gland – development and maintenance. Lactation, Vol I. Academic Press, New York

Sosa R, Kennell J H, Klaus M H, Urrutia J J 1976 The effect of early mother infant contact on breastfeeding, infection and growth. In Breastfeeding and the mother. Ciba Foundation Symposium 45. Elsevier, Amsterdam

Sousa P L R, Barros F C, Gazelle R V *et al* 1974 Attachment and lactation. In Proceedings of the 14th International Congress of Paediatricians, Buenos Aires, 1974

Stevens S, Whitfield M F 1980 How accurate is clinical test weighing of the newborn? Midwives Chronicle 93 (1108): 148–49

Stoppard M 1982 Your baby: 75–6. Octopus Books, London

Sutherland J M, Glueck H I, Gleser G 1967 Hemorrhagic disease of the newborn: breastfeeding as a necessary factor in the pathogenesis. American Journal of Diseases in Childhood 113: 524–33

Thomsen A C, Espersen T, Maigaard S 1984 Course and treatment of milk stasis, non-infectious inflammation of the breast and infectious mastitis in nursing women. American Journal of Obstetrics and Gynecology 149: 492–95

Thomson M E, Hartsock T G, Larson C 1979 The importance of immediate postnatal contact: its effect on breastfeeding. Canadian Family Physician 25: 1374–78

Tyson J E, Wang P H, Guyda H, Friesen H G 1977 Studies of prolactin secretion in human pregnancy. American Journal of Obstetrics and Gynecology 129: 454

von Kries R, Shearer M, McCarthy P T, Haug M, Harzer G, Gobel U 1987 Vitamin K1 content of maternal milk: influence of the stage of lactation, lipid composition and vitamin K1 supplements given to the mother. Paediatric Research 22: 513–17

Wahlberg V, Lungh W, Winberg J 1982 Reconsideration of Créde's prophylaxis: IV. Effects of silver nitrate on mother–infant relationship. Acta Paediatrica Scandinavica 295 (Supplement): 49–57

Whichelow M J 1982 Factors associated with the duration of breastfeeding in a privileged society. Early Human Development 7: 273–80

Whitehead R G, Paul A A 1981 Infant growth and human milk requirements. Lancet ii: 161–63

Whitehead R G, Paul A A, Black A E, Wiles S J 1981 Recommended dietary amount of energy for pregnancy or lactation in the UK. In Torun B, Young V R, Rang W M (eds) Protein energy requirement of developing countries: evaluation of new data: 259–65. United Nations University, Tokyo

Whitfield M F, Kay R, Stevens S 1981 Validity of routine clinical test weighing as a measure of the intake of breastfed babies. Archives of Diseases in Childhood 56: 919–21

Widstrom A M, Ransjo-Arvidson A B, Christensson H K, Mattiesen A S, Winberg J, Uvnas-Moberg K 1987 Gastric suction in healthy newborn infants: effects on circulation and developing feeding behaviour. Acta Paediatric Scandinavica 76: 566–72

Winberg J, Wesser G 1971 Does breastmilk protect against septicaemia in the newborn? Lancet i: 1091–94

Wood C S, Isaacs P C, Jensen M, Hilton H G 1988 Exclusively breastfed infants: growth and caloric intake. Paediatric Nursing 14: 117–25

Woolridge M W, Baum J D, Drewett R F 1980 Effect of a traditional and of a new nipple shield on sucking patterns and milk flow. Early Human Development 4: 357–64

Woolridge M W, Baum J D, Drewett R F 1982 Individual patterns of milk intake during breastfeeding. Early Human Development 7: 265–72

Woolridge M W, Greasley V, Silpiornkosol S 1985 The initiation of lactation: the effect of early versus delayed contact for suckling on milk intake in the first week postpartum. A study in Chiang Mai, Northern Thailand. Early Human Development   12: 269–78
Woolridge M W 1986a The anatomy of infant sucking. Midwifery   2: 164–71
Woolridge M W 1986b Aetiology of sore nipples. Midwifery   2: 172–6
Woolridge M, Fisher C 1988 Colic overfeeding and symptoms of lactose malabsorption in the breastfed baby: a possible artifact of feeding management? Lancet   ii: 382–84

■ Suggested further reading

Inch S, Garforth S 1989 Establishing and maintaining breastfeeding. In Chalmers I, Enkin M, Kierse M (eds) Effective care in pregnancy and childbirth: Chapter 80. Oxford University Press, Oxford
Inch S, Renfrew M J 1989 Common breastfeeding problems. In Chalmers I, Enkin M, Kierse M (eds) Effective care in pregnancy and childbirth: Chapter 81. Oxford University Press, Oxford
Inch S 1987 Difficulties with breastfeeding – midwives in disarray? Journal of the Royal Society of Medicine   80: 53–8
Minchin M 1985 Breastfeeding Matters. Alma Publications, Australia; Allen and Unwin, London
Palmer G 1988 The politics of breastfeeding. Pandora Press, Allen and Unwin, London
Woolridge M 1986 The anatomy of infant sucking. Midwifery   2: 164–71
Woolridge M 1986 The aetiology of sore nipples. Midwifery   2: 172–76
Woolridge M, Fisher C 1988 Colic 'overfeeding' and symptoms of lactose malabsorption in the breastfed baby: a possible artifact of feeding management? Lancet   382–84
Successful breastfeeding – a practical guide for midwives. Handbook produced by the Royal College of Midwives. Obtainable from the RCM, 15, Mansfield Street, London W1M 0BE

Chapter 3

Emotional problems associated with childbirth

Jenifer M Holden

This chapter discusses recent research which shows that, for many women, childbirth is not the joyful experience portrayed by the media, and examines the evidence that unresolved emotional problems at this time may have long-term implications not only for the woman herself, but for her whole family. It also outlines what professionals can do to help, including a rationale for counselling and social support.

Psychological disturbances associated with birth are not a recent phenomenon; they were first noted by the ancient Greek physicians and were recorded in detail in the nineteenth century by the French psychiatrists Marce and Esquirol. In the last few decades, however, although the physical risks associated with giving birth have been reduced considerably, technological advances leading to the increasing mechanisation of childbirth have contributed to a lessened emphasis on the emotional needs of individual women. Fortunately much has been achieved recently to bring back a more human perspective on this natural function, and there has been a renewed recognition among professionals that the emotional wellbeing of mothers both during and after delivery is extremely important. Women themselves, and the media, have also been instrumental in bringing about improvements as the changing role of women in society leads them to view marriage and childrearing as only one of their options. Having made a conscious decision to have a child, women are increasingly aware of their right to make choices in the way they give birth. They may also be less prepared to tolerate the disabling effects of postnatal depression than women of previous generations.

■ Before reading this chapter you should:

● Watch parents interacting with their baby;
● Read through the notes of someone who has suffered from postnatal depression.

■ Emotional disturbances associated with childbirth

Emotional problems after childbirth are usually classified into 'the blues', postnatal depression and puerperal psychosis. These distinctions may be blurred, however, as they are based mainly on the relative severity of the symptoms.

□ The blues

The blues is the name given to the rapid fluctuations in mood experienced by around 50–70 per cent of all mothers during the week or so following delivery. Elation may be followed by tears for apparently trivial reasons and, although most women recover their equanimity fairly quickly, some have more severe reactions. The frequent occurrence of the blues (and a lack of evidence for any association with psychosocial factors) suggests that it may have a biological cause, the dramatic change in hormone secretion level following delivery having being proposed as the most likely precipitating factor (Nott *et al* 1976). It may also be considered, however, as a reaction to the emotional and physical stress of giving birth. Many people experience emotional lability similar to the blues a few days after an operation.

Stein (1982) described two different components of the blues. The first is a distinct short-lasting episode, characterised by weeping, which occurs some time between the third and tenth day. The second is more severe and persistent, with a cluster of symptoms including depression, irritability, tension, confusion, anxiety, headache, restlessness, and insomnia, occurring in different combinations and varying severity in individual women. Stein suggested that these two components may have different causes, and that more severe cases of the blues may be the start of a longer lasting postnatal disturbance. As Kendell (1985) pointed out, the timing of the blues coincides with the timing of the onset of most puerperal psychoses, suggesting that whatever trigger mechanism is responsible for the blues may also precipitate psychosis in predisposed women.

Although the blues is so common as to be almost the norm, to every woman it is a unique experience. All women suffering from the blues should be treated with sympathy and understanding related to their individual needs, and those with severe symptoms should be closely monitored, and followed up after their return home from hospital.

□ Puerperal psychosis

At the other end of the scale is the much rarer puerperal psychosis. Although only two or three of every thousand women who give birth will develop a psychosis, this proportion is startlingly high when compared with the likelihood of psychiatric illness at other times of life. Paffenbarger (1964) found that 18 times more women were admitted to mental hospitals in the month following childbirth than at any other time in their life, and a study by Dean and Kendell in Edinburgh (1981) confirmed that there is a dramatic peak of psychiatric admissions at this time. Whether this increased incidence is due to a syndrome specific to the puerperium, or simply to more women being precipitated into psychosis by the stress of childbirth, is unclear.

The term 'psychosis' covers a range of conditions; women may present with depression, mania, delirium or delusions resembling schizophrenia. The onset in any individual is usually sudden and dramatic, with an obvious need for urgent treatment. The woman typically becomes very confused, suspicious, distrustful or even aggressive, showing a lack of contact with reality, and often expressing bizarre thoughts. For instance she may believe that someone is out to kill her, or she may want to kill someone herself. One mother saw it as her mission to kill the baby of a fellow patient, believing that it was a voodoo baby which was exerting an evil influence on her own child.

Specialist care is essential and women with psychoses have traditionally been treated in psychiatric hospitals. Progress has been made in recent years with the provision of special mother-and-baby units, but in areas lacking this facility women may be separated from their babies at a vulnerable time in the development of their relationship. In Nottingham community psychiatric liaison and intensive home nursing has made it possible for many psychotic women to be treated at home (Oates 1988) and it is hoped that this example will spread. With modern treatments, puerperal psychoses have an excellent prognosis and most women recover within two to three months (Cox 1986).

☐ **Postnatal depression**

> 'I enjoyed my pregnancy and I enjoyed having him, it was the greatest thing I have ever experienced until I came home. And then I thought, God, I don't want you.... I felt as if I was inside this box, all by myself, with nobody to help me, or to help me understand why I was like this.... I have been sad before and I have been unhappy, but never like after I had Thomas, to the point where I just didn't want to live any more.'

Susan was interviewed during a study in Edinburgh of counselling by health visitors in postnatal depression (Holden *et al* 1989). Her description of her feelings after giving birth to her first child will have a familiar ring to members of the caring professions who have close contact with mothers. Susan was happily married with no financial or housing worries, had planned her pregnancy, attended antenatal classes and looked forward eagerly to the birth of her baby. Why did she respond to motherhood in this way? Was her case unusual? Was she ill? Can anything be done to help women like Susan? These are questions which researchers over the past 20 years have been trying to answer.

Susan's unhappiness started shortly after she came home from hospital, and her symptoms fit into the category of 'non-psychotic postnatal depression', which falls between the blues and puerperal psychosis in severity. Postnatal depression is more severe and longer-lasting than the blues, but is less dramatic than psychosis, and so it is less easily recognised. As in Susan's case, this type of disturbance has a gradual onset and before six weeks after birth is not easy to distinguish from the fatigue and emotional lability experienced by most mothers as they recover from the delivery and adjust to the demands of the new baby.

In an influential study Brice Pitt (1968) found that 11 per cent of 330 women became depressed in the six weeks after delivery. Further studies showed a remarkably consistent prevalence, varying between 10 and 16 per cent (Cox et al 1982; Kumar & Robson 1984; Watson et al 1984). These studies also showed that many women continue to experience psychological problems for several months; some women were still depressed when interviewed four years after delivery. Women who become depressed postnatally are also more likely to have further depressive episodes, especially following subsequent deliveries. It is not clear whether this persistent susceptibility to depression is a direct consequence of postnatal depression or is due to a pre-existing vulnerability.

☐ **What is postnatal depression like?**

Although few women with postnatal depression require psychiatric help, the experience is deeply distressing. From interviews with his subjects Pitt made a synopsis of their symptoms. He found that their depression was characterised by:

> tearfulness, despondency, feelings of inadequacy and inability to cope, particularly with the baby ... self-reproach over not loving or caring enough for the baby ... excessive anxiety over the baby which was not justified by the babies' health .. Unusual irritability was common, sometimes adding to feelings of guilt ... impaired concentration and memory, and undue fatigue and ready exhaustion were frequent, so that mothers could barely deal with their babies, let alone look after the rest of the family and cope with housework and shopping .... Anorexia was present with remarkable consistence, and sleep disturbances, over and above that inevitable with a new baby, were reported by a third of the patients, taking the form of difficulty in getting off to sleep, rather than early morning waking (Pitt 1968).

This vivid description clearly reveals the suffering caused to the mother, and intimates possible effects on the mother-infant relationship which will be discussed later. The symptoms of postnatal depression vary in individual women, but the most important indication is a change in the mother's normal character and behaviour. Descriptions of their experience given by women who took part in the Edinburgh counselling study (Holden *et al* 1989) show how unusual their symptoms seemed even to themselves:

> 'I have never felt like that in my life before. Nobody could speak to me because I would burst into tears at the least thing. I took an extreme dislike to everybody in this world except my baby. I wanted everybody to go away, I was interested in nothing.'

> 'It was terrible. It was like someone else taking over. I wasn't the same person any more. I didn't recognise myself. It wasn't me, that was what I kept saying. It wasn't me.'

> 'It was absolutely ghastly. It felt as if there was a physical weight inside that was dragging me down. I was pulling it around all the time, and everything was an effort.'

■ Effects of maternal depression on children

Depression after childbirth is not only traumatic for the mother, but can affect the whole quality of family life and there are strong indications that it may have effects on the intellectual, social and emotional development of children. Rutter (1979) observed that important influences on a child's early cognitive development are the provision by parents of a variety of activities and opportunities for play and conversation, and responsiveness to the child's signals. Trevarthen (1980) showed that the development of communication skills is largely dependent on the mother's ability to respond closely to cues from her infant.

Lynne Murray (1988) reported on a study examining videotaped interactions of mothers with their babies. She has found that some depressed mothers (particularly those for whom this was their first experience of depression) are less responsive to their infant's social signals than nondepressed mothers. Infants typically respond to a lack of response in their mother by showing distress or withdrawal. Murray suggested that patterns of behaviour may be set up in the baby which may persist even when the mother has recovered and is able to respond affectionately, and that this may limit their subsequent experience. Those babies whose mothers were less responsive to their signals were found to perform less well on developmental tasks at nine months.

Other researchers have found evidence for problems in the children of mothers whose depression appeared to be related to childbirth. Cogill *et al* (1986) found significant intellectual deficits in four-year-olds whose mothers had suffered depression during the first year of the child's life, and Richman (1978) reported that 75 per cent of a sample of children with reading difficulties at age eight had mothers who were depressed when the child was three. Wrate *et al* (1985) found behavioural problems in the three-year-old children of mothers who had had postnatal depressive episodes.

Depression may affect the quality of the relationship between mother and child. Robson and Kumar (1980) found that mothers who were depressed three months after delivery were more likely to express dislike or indifference towards their babies, while Uddenberg and Englesson (1978) found that depressed mothers tended to describe their four and a half-year old child in a negative way. (Interestingly enough, the children also described their mothers more negatively than did the children of non-depressed mothers.) It may also be true, however, that babies have an effect on their mother's mood. Cutrona and Troutman (1986) found that infant temperamental difficulty was strongly related to the mother's level of depression at three months after delivery. The research evidence would therefore seem to indicate that depression in mothers is frequently associated with problems in their children.

■ Relationship with the partner

It is gradually being recognised that becoming parents can in itself affect the relationship between the couple. Moss *et al* (1987) found that for more than one in ten couples the transition to parenthood had serious adverse consequences on their relationship, younger couples and those with shorter relationships being most affected. Clearly childbirth can be stressful for both parents; O'Hara *et al* (1985) found that depression increased in both husband and wife during pregnancy and after delivery, and that depressed women tended to have depressed partners. Wolkind *et al* (1980) expressed concern about the possibility of husbands being ill-prepared for the loss of closeness caused by the arrival of a baby, particularly the first. They may be even less prepared for the alienation which may result from depression in their partner. Pitt (1968) described the intense irritability directed particularly towards the spouse; this may be interpreted by the husband as hostility rather than an indication that his partner needs help, as can be seen from this quotation from an interview with the partner of one of the women who took part in the Edinburgh counselling study (Holden *et al* 1989):

> 'It is terrible, no matter what you do, you are wrong. She is awfully quick tempered, things that normally she would laugh about, she doesn't. She has changed an awful lot. You sometimes say to yourself ... is she tired of me? Is she sick of me? Well, you do.'

Pregnancy, birth and child care were traditionally regarded as the mother's role, fathers being responsible for providing the material needs of the family. For Winnicot (1957) it was enough that the father should 'be alive and stay alive during his child's early years'. This view is changing but, although fathers increasingly expect to take a more active role in child care, research evidence suggests that most men do not yet take an equal role in parenting. Beail (1985) found that although fathers will play with their baby, walk a crying baby or feed it during the day, they are less keen to participate in nappy changing or night feeds. Nor, it seems, do men take an equal share in domestic chores. Moss *et al* (1987) found that 'there is no sign that the basic structure of the sexual division of labour has been significantly redesigned. Help is given when it is asked for, not as a matter of course'. Paykel *et al* (1980) found that lack of help from the partner was associated with postnatal depression; husbands of depressed women did significantly less in the way of household chores, shopping and sharing the care of other children than those of non-depressed women. There is, however, evidence that if fathers are encouraged during pregnancy to take a more active role they will do so, and that this has an effect on the reaction of their partner to the stress of mothering. For example, Gordon *et al* (1965) found that women who were encouraged during pregnancy to confide in their husband and enlist his practical help did get more help and were less likely to be depressed after delivery.

■ Why do some women have emotional problems after having a baby?

□ Psychosocial factors

On the whole, research findings suggest that factors associated with emotional disturbance after childbirth apply equally to vulnerability at other times of life. For example, most studies show that having had previous depression (especially following the birth of a baby) increases the likelihood of a recurrence, as does a family psychiatric history. Brown and Harris (1978) showed that stressful life events contribute to depression; and several researchers have found this to be true for depression after childbirth (Paykel *et al* 1980; Watson *et al* 1984; O'Hara 1985). Birth itself is stressful, and new mothers may be particularly vulnerable to events such as bereavement, a family crisis, loss of a job, a change of house; or to chronic problems, such as poor housing, financial worries or even bad relationships with neighbours. Depression may be a grief response to a recent loss, or the birth of the new baby may reawaken unresolved grief for a previous distressing event such as a miscarriage, termination of pregnancy or stillbirth. The onset of depression can often coincide with the realisation that one is in an inescapable situation; childbirth may represent such a situation for women who were ambivalent about having the baby, or for those who already have other small children to care for.

Whether individuals have an adverse response to stressful events depends to a large extent on whether or not they see themselves as being able to exercise control over their life. The feeling that one is unable to influence one's circumstances leads to a condition known as 'learned helplessness' (Seligman 1975). Women may feel helpless (and become depressed) in adverse social circumstances which they cannot change; for example having a baby may mean that a woman with no income is unable to take a job.

□ Hormonal factors

To date there is no research showing a direct association between hormonal changes and the onset of non-psychotic depression, although some support for a hormonal link comes from a study which looked at the relationship of breastfeeding, oral contraceptives and postnatal depression. Alder and Cox (1983) found that women who were totally breastfeeding and not on the pill were the most likely group to experience symptoms of depression at 3–5 months postpartum. Interestingly enough, those who were not on the pill but were only partially breastfeeding had the lowest risk of depression. There are both physiological and psychosocial explanations for this apparent paradox; women who are fully breastfeeding have lower oestrogen levels, associated with loss of libido and vaginal dryness. This in itself can lead to a lack of closeness with the partner; love-making may also be less enjoyable due to exhaustion and the likelihood of being interrupted by a hungry baby who can only be fed by his weary mum. A baby who has the odd bottle or solid feed can be handed over occasionally, but total breast-feeders have little time off from their baby and, depending on the attitudes of their friends and family and the amount of available help, may find it takes longer to resume their social life. While many women find deep fulfillment in their baby's total dependence, realising that this precious time is not for ever, it does inevitably mean a loss of personal freedom. In Western society, breastfeeding is not socially acceptable everywhere, neither are feeding mothers accorded special status or privileges.

It is obviously important that women are encouraged to get in touch with how they feel about breastfeeding, before and after birth, and feel free to make an informed choice, on the basis of their own needs as well as those of the baby. Those who decide to fully breastfeed may need extra counselling and support.

■ Relationships past and present

Vulnerability to emotional problems starts with early experiences, and having been loved, valued and understood by those closest to us in childhood is perhaps the strongest protection against emotional disturbance. The responsibility of mothering a baby may seem less awesome to someone who has had a satisfying experience of being nurtured herself. Frommer and O'Shea (1973) considered the effect of parental deprivation in childhood on mothering. Women who reported being separated from one or both parents before the age of 11 had a higher incidence of depression and were more anxious about their babies than non-separated women. The present relationship with one's own mother (or carer) is also important. A mother who is also a friend can be a great source of support after childbirth, especially if she continues to mother her daughter rather than bypassing her to mother the baby. Women who do not have a supportive mother (or a nurturing substitute) may be in need of extra support.

☐ **Confiding relationships**

Brown and Harris (1978) and Campbell *et al* (1983) found that women who had an intimate confiding relationship were less likely to become depressed, and having a confidant has been shown to protect women against postnatal depression (Cutrona and Troutman 1986). Simply being married or having a partner does not guarantee having someone in whom to confide; many of the women who took part in the Edinburgh counselling study (Holden *et al* 1989) said that although their partner was supportive in practical ways, they found it difficult to talk to him about their feelings. Several studies have shown an association between lack of confiding or actual disharmony in the marital relationship and postnatal depression. Paykel *et al* (1980), who rated women's perception of the extent to which they could tell their partner their worries and problems and the extent to which he would listen or avoid, found that depressed women had significantly worse ratings than controls.

■ **Conclusions**

A multifactorial explanation is attractive, childbirth being seen as the final stress factor for women whose nature and past experience have already rendered them vulnerable, or who have a number of recent or current stressors. Childbirth is *not* just another stressor however. Becoming a mother involves physical experiences including pain and exhaustion, and a whole gamut of emotions including excitement, apprehension, fear, relief, joy and love. It also means accepting responsibility for the wellbeing of a totally dependent and relatively helpless human being for twenty four hours a day. The onset of 'postnatal depression' may simply mean that the realisation of this responsibility becomes overwhelming, especially to someone who lacks emotional or practical support for themselves.

■ Implications

The literature clearly shows that the period immediately following child-birth is of critical importance in the establishment of the relationship between mother and baby, and of the family as a harmonious and successfully functioning unit. The implications of emotional disturbance at this time for the mother herself are sufficient to merit special attention. If we also take into consideration the long-term effects of the other's psychological health on the family, it can be seen that the early diagnosis and active treatment of emotional problems associated with childbirth should be a matter of the highest priority.

☐ Physical treatments

Although antidepressants are a useful treatment for severe or persistent depression, Kumar and Robson (1984) and Cox (1986) agreed that clearer guidelines are needed about the contraindications for prescribing psychotropic drugs for pregnant and lactating women. Snaith (1983) pointed out that haste in prescribing medical treatments for postnatal depression should be avoided, and that benzodiazepines in particular can lead to increased irritability which may convert a potential into an actual baby batterer. Some physical treatments have been found to have a useful preventive function. Diana Riley (1986) found less depression at one month and one year following delivery in women treated with pyridoxine (vitamin B_6). Katharina Dalton (1980) believes that there is a direct connection between premenstrual tension and postnatal depression. For high-risk women she prescribes progesterone injections from the onset of labour and then daily for eight days, followed by progesterone suppositories until the return of menstruation. This treatment, however, has yet to be tested in a double-blind placebo trial.

☐ Social support

Oakley (1988) pointed out in a literature review that there is strong evidence that social support can benefit the health of both mothers and babies. Social support encompasses both practical and emotional support, and may include counselling and education, or even research programmes which result in the mother feeling that extra interest is being shown in her welfare.

☐ Antenatal support

There is evidence that antenatal education programmes which include a social support component (or which provide conditions which are conducive to the promotion of self help support) are of most benefit in reducing problems postnatally. Hillier and Slade (1989), who assessed women before and after attending antenatal classes, found that while confidence in coping with labour and caring for the newborn infant increased following both hospital and community based classes, the latter had the advantage of promoting supportive social relationships. Elliott *et al* (1988) found that women who were invited to informal groups which started antenatally and provided information about the realities of parenthood, including the possibility of postnatal depression, showed only half the prevalence of depression found in a group of randomly selected noninvited mothers. The support provided by these groups came only partly from the input from professionals; the women themselves took over the running of the group which continued to meet postnatally. There is some evidence, however, that professional intervention is more helpful; in a randomised controlled trial Barnett and Parker (1986) found a 19 per cent reduction in anxiety during the first postnatal year in a group of highly anxious primiparous mothers who received professional help – compared to a 12 per cent reduction in women who received support from nonprofessionals. (Women who received no intervention at all showed only a 3 per cent reduction in anxiety).

Antenatal education can also help relationships after delivery; Sheresefsky and Lockman (1973) showed that marital relationships of women who were given antenatal counselling about the possible effect of childbirth on the relationship remained stable, whereas those in a control group had deteriorated by six months postpartum.

☐ **Social support and delivery**

The many studies which are concerned with psychological aspects of delivery, and with the importance of involving women in decisions about their confinement, have been amply chronicled elsewhere (for example Leboyer 1975; Kitzinger 1978; Oakley 1981; Odent 1984; Ball 1987). In this chapter it is sufficient to say that emotional support can significantly affect the outcome of labour. Enlightening studies by Sosa *et al* (1980) and Klaus *et al* (1986) showed that the provision of a supportive non-professional person who stayed with the mother throughout childbirth not only reduced the time of labour by half, but dramatically reduced complications for both mother and baby. There is some evidence that the woman's perception of the emotional support provided by her companion is an important factor. Henneborn and Cogan (1975) reported that women's satisfaction with birth was enhanced by the presence of their partner, and that accompanied women had less painful deliveries. In contrast, women in a study by Melzack (1984) reported more pain when the partner was present, and in *Birth Reborn*, Odent (1984) commented that the partner's presence may not always be beneficial. Niven (1985) studied the experience of parturient women, most of whom were accompanied by their partner during labour. The majority of the accompanied women said that their partner's presence enhanced their experience; they also reported less pain than women who did not find their partner's presence helpful and than the women who had no companion. Some women who did not find their partner's presence helpful said that they had been concerned that he might be distressed by witnessing the birth or by their pain. Niven concluded that, 'the mere presence of a birth companion is not necessarily perceived by the parturant as positive, and the decision to be present should be made by the couple in the light of their knowledge of each other and of the woman's coping style'.

☐ **Postnatal support and counselling**

In *Reactions to Motherhood* Jean Ball (1987) concluded that, 'the person experiencing stress can be helped by someone whose unconditional support is available to them'. This view is shared by many. Snaith (1983) maintained that for the majority of distressed mothers the most useful treatment is explanation, understanding and support, and similar observations were made by Bichard *et al* (1985), Kumar and Robson (1984) and Cox (1986). Counselling would seem to be the ideal first line of treatment for women with emotional problems after childbirth. A counsellor not only acts as a professional confidant, but can also provide social support. In a randomised controlled trial in Edinburgh, health visitors were given a brief training in nondirective counselling and asked to pay eight counselling visits at weekly intervals to women who had been identified as depressed by a psychiatrist. A control group of similarly depressed women did not receive the extra visits. After three months when the women were reassessed by the psychiatrist (who did not know to which group the women had been assigned) two thirds of the counselled mothers had recovered from their depression, compared with only one third of depressed mothers in the control group (Holden *et al* 1989). The therapeutic value of talking to an empathic listener was clear from comments made by the women in separate tape recorded interviews after the second diagnosis had been recorded. For example, Kathy said:

> 'I talked to my health visitor about how I felt, and she just listened. When you articulate something, it makes you think about it. It helps to sort things out, and lets you see how small they are. It made me feel better that way.'

■ **Recommendations for clinical practice in the light of currently available evidence**

The main aim of clinical practice with regard to the psychological aspects of childbirth should be to create a climate in which women, their partners, and those involved in their care feel free to discuss the realities of parenthood, in which sufficient time is set aside for the discussion of emotional issues, and which provides or leads to the promotion of social support.

☐ 1. Antenatal preparation

Partners should be welcomed to the sessions and provided with information about how they can provide emotional as well as practical support. A fact sheet about postnatal depression should also be made available. Apart from preparation for the birth and infant care, this should include information about:

- The stresses involved in parenting;
- The possible effect of having a baby on the relationship between the couple;
- The importance of asking for help from the partner, and from others such as relatives or neighbours;
- The advantages of talking about one's feelings with one's partner or a close friend or professional;
- The possibility of adverse emotional responses after delivery, and available sources of help.

Where possible, classes should be held close to the woman's home, with an informal atmosphere, tea and biscuits, and encouragement to maintain a continuing support group after the baby is born. (See also the chapter on 'Antenatal education' by Tricia Murphy-Black in the volume in this series on *Antenatal Care*.)

☐ 2. In the postnatal ward and at home

Women's emotional responses should be closely monitored in the post-delivery period and staffing levels should be sufficient to allow midwives to spend up to half an hour of 'quality listening time' with each mother every day, ensuring that she is given explicit encouragement to talk fully about her feelings and about her experience of giving birth. Empathetic listening may not only be therapeutic in itself, but will facilitate the early recognition of women with problems. It is also possible that being encouraged to talk about their feelings in the early postnatal period may help to prevent later emotional problems from developing.

The blues should not be dismissed as 'normal'; in severe cases depression or psychosis may develop. In cases of obvious disturbance, a medical opinion will in any case be sought, but the health visitor and GP should be informed about any woman whose emotional equilibrium is not fully restored before she leaves the midwife's care.

■ Practice check

● How much time do you normally spend in constructive listening?

● How effective are you at encouraging women to talk about their feelings?

● During the next month, count the number of women in your care with the blues. Can you recognise the two components described by Stein (1982) on p 46 of this text?

● Can you find any differences between women who experience the blues and those who do not?

● In listening to one woman talking about her response to the experience of birth, how many separate emotions can you identify?

■ References

Alder E M, Cox J L 1983 Breastfeeding and postnatal depression. Journal of Psychosomatic Research 27: 139–44

Ball J 1987 Reactions to motherhood. Cambridge University Press, Cambridge

Barnett B, Parker G 1986 Possible determinants, correlates and consequences of high levels of anxiety in primiparous mothers. Psychological Medicine 16: 177–85

Beail N 1985 Fathers and infant caretaking. Journal of Reproductive and Infant Psychology 3 (2): 54–64

Bichard D et al 1985 Support, listen and love ... (three mothers' accounts of postnatal depression). New Generation (December): 46–8

Brown G W, Harris T 1978 Social origins of depression. Tavistock Publications, London

Campbell E, Cope S J, Teasdale J D 1983 Social factors and affective disorder: an investigation of the Brown and Harris model. British Journal of Psychiatry 143: 548–53

Cogill S R, Caplan H L, Alexandra H, Robson K R, Kumar R 1986 Impact of maternal postnatal depression on the cognitive development of young children. British Medical Journal 292: 1165–67

Cox J L 1986 Postnatal depression: a guide for health professionals. Churchill Livingstone, Edinburgh

Cox J L, Connor Y, Kendell R E 1982 Prospective study of the psychiatric disorders of childbirth. British Journal of Psychiatry 140: 111–17

Cutrona C E, Troutman B R 1986 Social support, infant temperament and parenting self-efficacy: a mediational model of postpartum depression. Child Development 57 (6): 1507–18

Dalton K 1980 Depression after childbirth. Oxford University Press, Oxford

Dean C, Kendell R E 1981 The symptomatology of puerperal illnesses. British Journal of Psychiatry 139: 128–33

Eliott S A, Sanjak M, Leverton T 1988 Parents' groups in pregnancy: a preventive intervention for postnatal depression? In Gottlieb B H (ed) Marshalling social support: formats, processes and effects. Sage Publications, London

Frommer E A, O'Shea G 1973 Antenatal identification of women liable to have problems in managing their infants. British Journal of Psychiatry 123: 149–56

Gordon E, Kapostins E E, Gordon K K 1965 Factors in postpartum emotional adjustment. Obstetrics and Gynaecology 25: 158–66

Henneborn W, Cogan R 1975 The effect of husband participation on reported pain and probability of medication during labour and birth. Journal of Psychosomatic Research 20: 15–22

Hillier C A, Slade P 1989 The impact of antenatal classes on knowledge, anxiety and confidence in primiparous women. Journal of Reproductive and Infant Psychology 7 (1): 3–15

Holden J M 1985 Talking it out. Nursing Times (Community Outlook, October) 81: 8–10

Holden J M 1986 Counselling for health visitors. In Cox J L Postnatal depression: a guide for health professionals. Churchill Livingstone, Edinburgh

Holden J M 1988 Banishing the blues. Nursing Times 84 (17): 31–2

Holden J M 1989 Health visitors in the front line. Edinburgh Medicine 56: 14–16

Holden J M, Sagovsky R, Cox L J 1989 Counselling in a general practice setting: a controlled study of health visitor intervention in the treatment of postnatal depression. British Medical Journal 298: 223–26

Kendell R E 1985 Emotional and physical factors in the genesis of mental disorders. Journal of Psychosomatic Research 29 (1): 3–11

Kitzinger S 1978 Women as mothers. Martin Robertson, Oxford

Klaus M H, Kennell J H, Robertson S S, Sosa R 1986 Effects of social support during parturition on maternal and infant morbidity. British Medical Journal 6: 585–87

Kumar R, Robson K M 1984 A prospective study of emotional disorders in child-bearing women. British Journal of Psychiatry 144: 35–47

Leboyer F 1975 Birth without violence. Wildwood House, London

Melzack R 1984 The myth of painless childbirth (John J Bonica Lecture). Pain 19: 321–37

Moss P, Bolland G, Foxman R, Owen C 1987 The division of household work during the transition to parenthood. Journal of Reproductive and Infant Psychology 5 (2): 71–87

Murray L 1988 Effects of postnatal depression on infant development: the contribution of direct studies of early mother-infant interaction. In Kumar R, Brockington I (eds) Motherhood and mental illness, Volume 2. John Wright, London

Niven K 1985 How helpful is the presence of the husband at childbirth? Journal of Reproductive and Infant Psychology   3 (2): 45–53

Nott P N, Franklin M, Armitage C, Gelder M G 1976 Hormonal changes in mood in the puerperium. British Journal of Psychiatry   128: 379–83

Oakley A 1988 Is social support good for the health of mothers and babies? Journal of Reproductive and Infant Psychology   6 (1): 3–23

Oakley A 1981 From here to maternity. Pelican, Harmondsworth

Oates M 1988 The development of an integrated community-oriented service for severe postnatal illness. In Kumar R, Brockington I F (eds) Motherhood and mental illness Vol 2. Causes and consequences. John Wright, London

Odent M 1984 Birth reborn. Souvenir Press, London

O'Hara M W, Rehm L P, Campbell S B 1982 Predicting depressive symptomatology; cognitive-behavioural models and postpartum depression. Journal of Abnormal Psychology   91: 457–61

O'Hara, M W, Neunaber D J, Zekoski E M 1984 Prospective study of postpartum depression: prevalence, course and predictive factors. Journal of Abnormal Psychology   93: 158–71

O'Hara M W 1985 Depression and marital adjustment during pregnancy and after delivery. American Journal of Family Therapy   4: 49–55

Paffenbarger R S 1964 Epidemiological aspects of postpartum mental illness. British Journal of Preventive Social Medicine   18: 189–95

Paykel E S, Emms E, Fletcher J, Rassaby E S 1980 Life events and social support in puerperal depression. British Journal of Psychiatry   136: 339–46

Pitt B 1968 Atypical depression following childbirth. British Journal of Psychiatry   114: 1325–35

Richman N 1978 Depression in mothers of young children. Journal of the Royal Society of Medicine   71: 489–93

Riley D 1986 An audit of obstetric liaison psychiatry in 1984. Journal of Reproductive and Infant Psychology   4: 99–115

Robson K M, Kumar R 1980 Delayed onset of maternal affection after childbirth. British Journal of Psychiatry   136: 347–53

Rutter M 1979 Protective factors in children's responses to stress and disadvantage. In Kent M W, Rolf J (eds) Primary prevention of psychopathology, Vol III. Social competence in children: 49–74. University Press of New England, Hanover, N H

Seligman E 1975 Helplessness: on depression, development and death. Freeman, San Francisco

Sheresefsky P M, Lockman R F 1973 Comparison of counseled and non-counseled groups. In Sheresefsky P M, Yarrow L J (eds) Psychological aspects of a first pregnancy: 151–63. Raven Press, New York

Snaith R P 1983 Pregnancy-related psychiatric disorder. British Journal of Hospital medicine   29 (5): 450–57

Sosa R, Kennell J R, Klaus M, Urruta J 1980 The effect of a supportive companion on perinatal problems, length of labour and mother-infant interaction. New England Journal of Medicine   303: 597–600

Stein G S 1982 The maternity blues. In Brockington I, Kumar C (eds) Motherhood and mental illness. Academic Press, London

Trevarthen C B 1980 Communication and cooperation in early infancy: a description of primary intersubjectivity. In Bullowa M (ed) Before speech. Cambridge University Press, Cambridge

Uddenberg N, Englesson I 1978 Prognosis of postpartum mental disturbance: prospective study of primiparous women and their four-and-a-half year old children. Acta Psychiatrica Scandinavica 58 (3): 201–12

Watson J P, Elliott S A, Rugg A J, Brough D I 1984 Psychiatric disorder in pregnancy and the first postnatal year. British Journal of Psychiatry 144: 453–62

Winnicot D W 1957 The child and the family: first relationships. Tavistock Publications, London

Wolkind S, Zajicek E, Ghodsian M 1980 Continuities in maternal depression. International Journal of Family Psychiatry 1: 167–82

Wrate R M, Rooney A C, Thomas P F, Cox J L 1985 Postnatal depression and child development: a 3-year follow-up study. British Journal of Psychiatry 146: 622–27

■ Suggested further reading

Ball J 1987 Reactions to Motherhood. Cambridge University Press, Cambridge

Cox J L 1986 Postnatal depression: a guide for health professionals. Churchill Livingstone, Edinburgh

Cox J L, Holden J M, Sagovsky R 1987 Detection of postnatal depression: development of the Edinburgh Postnatal Depression Scale. British Journal of Psychiatry 150: 782–86

Dainow S, Bailey C 1988 Developing skills with people: training for person to person client contact. John Wiley, Chichester

Holden J M 1989 A randomised controlled trial of counselling by health visitors in the treatment of postnatal depression. MPhil thesis, Faculty of Medicine, University of Edinburgh

Holden J M 1990 Postnatal depression: the health visitor as counsellor. In Faulkner A, Murphy-Black T (eds) Excellence in nursing: the research route: midwifery. Scutari Press, London

Nurse G 1980 Counselling and the nurse: an introduction. HM & M, Aylesbury

Oakley A 1981 From here to maternity. Pelican, Harmondsworth

Chapter 4

Parental–infant attachment

Ellena Salariya

In 1972, Klaus and colleagues described a 'sensitive period' occurring between a mother and her infant soon after birth which enhanced maternal-infant attachment. Interpretations applied to this suggestion evolved as the 'bonding theory' and affected midwifery practice in the delivery of care to mothers and babies throughout the Western world. Present practices, however, would appear to be based on the belief that if certain procedures are carried out during pregnancy, labour, delivery and in the postnatal period, satisfactory maternal-infant attachment will automatically follow. Caution must be exercised in believing this as several factors may contribute to mother-infant interaction and subsequent attachment which are beyond the control or understanding of professional care givers.

Childhood problems of behaviour, emotional deprivation, child abuse and neglect are thought to be related to problems of parenting and are responsible for a great proportion of morbidity in children. 'Interventions which increase the competence of parents and improve their sensitivity to their children, can be expected to decrease the occurrence of these problems' (Liptak *et al* 1983).

This chapter will examine attachment theory and consider what is thought to contribute to or detract from satisfactory maternal-infant interaction in the early neonatal period. The role of the midwife as an observer of early maternal care-giving is also discussed and her contribution in identifying which maternal-infant relationships are 'at risk' is postulated.

■ It is assumed that you are already aware of the following:

- National statistics, and how your local position compares with that in the country as a whole, in relation to:

- unemployment,
- quality of housing,
- single parent families,
- termination of pregnancy rate,
- divorce,
- drug and alcohol abuse,
- 'at risk' registered children,
- incidence of child abuse.

● The nuclear versus the extended family situation should be appreciated in relation to facilitating attachment. You may also be able to discuss relationships and attachment within your own family experience.

■ Bonding and attachment

Bonding and attachment are terms used in relation to aspects of affectionate relationships which develop between mother and child, father and child or others at differing times in the child's development. Bonding is usually considered to be the early one-way affection felt by a mother for her infant soon after delivery (Klaus & Kennell 1976) while attachment is recognised as a two-way interaction between a child and his mother or other person, and develops during the first year of life.

A 'critical period' has been described as important to the attachment mechanism for imprinting in birds (Bowlby 1969). Hess (1973) maintains that a similar critical period exists for the human species, when attachment is facilitated between a mother and her baby, very soon after birth. Other researchers (Hales *et al* 1977; Klaus *et al* 1972) prefer to use 'sensitive period' for human attachment timing, believing that mothers can form attachments to their infants up to and beyond three days after delivery. Klaus and Kennell (1976) proposed that separation between a mother and her infant in the first three days of life adversely affects the mother-child relationship and should be avoided. It has also been suggested that the quality of early mother-child relationships can affect the long-term experience of the child.

□ Attachment

Attachment has been defined as 'an enduring and unique emotional relationship between two people which is specific and endures through time' (Kennell *et al* 1975). Maternal attachment has been further defined by Robson and Powell (1982) as having three main elements:

- That the mother has a strong affection for her baby;
- That the affection will endure over time;
- That she has an awareness of her baby's needs and will respond appropriately.

The role of care-giver is considered complementary to attachment and implies that the person:

> is available and responsive as and when wanted, and is able to intervene judiciously should the child being cared for be heading for trouble.   (Bowlby 1977)

☐ **Early maternal contact and attachment**

The effects of early extended maternal-infant contact have been examined in several studies (Klaus *et al* 1972; Hales *et al* 1977; de Chateau and Wiberg 1977). In early extended contact, mothers are permitted to handle their infants soon after delivery for extra and/or longer periods of time than is usual hospital policy. The studies demonstrated that mothers engaged in more affectionate behaviours such as fondling, kissing, speaking, touching and looking en face (a position in which the mother aligns her head in the same parallel plane of rotation as the infant). At follow-up mothers were reported to be more reluctant to leave their infants with babysitters and were more interested in the paediatrician's physical examination of the baby.

More recently, Anisfeld and Lipper (1983) examined the effects of social support in relation to early contact and mother/infant bonding. The results demonstrated that early contact mothers smiled and spoke significantly more to their infants and they kissed and attempted to elicit a response from their babies more than did the later contact group. The most significant finding of the study demonstrated that women with high social support showed the same amount of affectionate behaviour, whether or not they received the early contact with their infant. By contrast, women with low social support who did not receive early contact, interacted minimally with their infants. Those who also received low support but had experienced early contact with their infants exhibited affectionate behaviour when looking at the infant (en face), smiling, vocalising, touching (other than that necessary to support the infant), kissing, stroking, rocking, inspecting and attempting to elicit a response from the infant.

The authors speculate that women with low social support are probably more likely to benefit from early infant contact. As it is not possible to determine which mothers are more in need of this as they arrive for delivery, they suggest that it would seem prudent to offer early maternal/infant contact to all. Other writers (Campbell & Taylor 1980) are critical, however, of the growing enthusiasm for early mother-child contact in the hope of long-lasting benefits for the child and suggest that there is little evidence to support such an hypothesis. Parents who wished for but were unable to enjoy early contact with their infant, should be counselled 'that early contact, although pleasant and desirable, is in no way essential for optimal bonding and subsequent satisfactory relationships' (Campbell & Taylor 1980). It would not be unrealistic to assume that the majority of readers of this textbook did not experience early maternal contact and are testimony to the fact that they have not been adversely affected by such 'deprivation'.

In a review of the maternal-infant relationship literature Goldberg (1983) also suggests that the existence of a 'sensitive period' is neither proven nor denied. It is unfortunate that the adjectives 'critical' and 'sensitive' have been misinterpreted by both professional and lay personnel in relation to early maternal/child contact. The newly delivered mother who is separated from her baby at the time of his birth may always believe that the opportunity to 'bond' with her infant was lost. Midwives should be aware of such a misconception and offer counselling as suggested by Campbell and Taylor earlier.

☐ **Early paternal contact and attachment**

Until about 20 years ago, the role of the father was very limited at and around the time of birth. Facilities were unavailable for 'expectant' fathers to attend parentcraft classes or to be present throughout their partners' labour and delivery. The father usually saw his infant through a viewing window several hours after birth. The baby was 'swaddled' and held by a midwife for this very brief encounter at a distance of around 24 inches. In some hospitals, babies remained at the 'bottom' of the mother's bed during day-time hours after the first two or three days and were returned to the nursery at night. The mothers were not encouraged to respond to their infants' cues and were expected to call a 'midwife' if and when the baby required attention.

Visiting hours also necessitated the removal of the cots from the ward area although in some 'avant garde' maternity units, the babies were left at the 'bedside' for the fathers' visiting hour.

The 'lying-in period' for women at this time was around 7–10 days for spontaneous or instrumental deliveries and 14 days if a caesarean section had been performed. While maternal–infant interaction was limited, father–infant interaction remained almost non-existent and sibling interaction impossible during the period of hospitalisation of mother and baby.

It was hypothesised by Parke and O'Leary (1976) that opportunities for early interaction with the infant may be especially important for father–infant attachment because fathers, they thought, might not be biologically or culturally primed to be responsive to infant cues. A study by Keller *et al* (1985) found that fathers given four hours extra contact with their infants during the neonatal period were more positive about their father–infant relationship than fathers who had not experienced extra contact at this time. Both groups of fathers had attended parentcraft classes and were present at the delivery of their baby. The results demonstrated more similarities than differences in the two groups however and the researchers recommended that further work should focus on what actually transpires between infants and their parents during early contact.

Early paternal-infant attachment was described by Greenberg and Morris (1974) as 'engrossment'. They proposed that 'engrossment' described self esteem and self worth in the father as a result of being present at the birth. The father in turn demonstrated more interest and affection towards the baby. In another study fathers were found to evidence more 'en face' behaviour with their infants after being present at the baby's birth compared to fathers who did not attend the delivery (Bower & Miller 1980).

The viewing of a 15 minute instructional videotape by fathers during the postnatal period also had positive effects on the degree of involvement the fathers had with their newborn infants. The video demonstrated different abilities of the newborn as well as care-taking techniques (Boyd 1981).

☐ **Early care giving**

In hospital before the 1970s, maternal–child contact, early or extended, was not considered by midwives or doctors to be a priority at or around the time of childbirth. After delivery, the baby was wrapped in a towel and blanket and quickly taken off to the ward nursery to be weighed, bathed and clothed. The mother may have been afforded a cursory glance at her infant's face prior to his removal and would see him several hours later, according to hospital policy.

Hospital personnel concentrated upon providing high quality physical care, always conscious of the need to prevent the spread of infection. This may have determined the infrequent interaction permitted between a mother and her baby during the puerperal/neonatal period in British maternity wards at this time. Mothers were allowed only limited interaction during feeding sessions, the infant being brought from the nursery at four-hourly intervals for either breast or bottle feeding. All care was carried out away from the mother's view and included daily bathing, umbilical cord care, weighing and four-hourly nappy changing, before and after each feed.

Infant bathing was demonstrated to the mother one day before her transfer home from hospital and she could bath her own baby, under supervision, before leaving. Midwives had been conditioned to believe that mothers were probably 'not their infants' best friends' relative to cross infection and we understood this to be the reason for the enforced separation of mother and child at this time.

☐ Mother–child relationships

The importance of mother-child relationships had been demonstrated by earlier writers who recognised the effects of maternal deprivation in children who had experienced periodic or total separation from their mothers before five years of age (Bowlby 1951; Schaffer & Emerson 1964; Ainsworth 1962).

Newborn infants were assumed to be too immature to be influenced by their environment or were thought to be passive recipients of in-coming stimuli such as food and warmth. It had been suggested that babies bonded to those who fed them but this was refuted by Winnicott (1968) who found that infants also attached to later care givers who had not nurtured them. Schaffer and Emerson (1964) found that although mothers tended to be the main feeders of infants, the main attachment figure for half the children in this study was not the mother but 30 per cent father and 20 per cent other (for example, siblings). This early 'thinking' may have influenced the behaviour of nursing personnel in hospital in the belief that 'anyone could feed and give care to the neonate' and that separation from his mother in a ward nursery 'could not possibly do him any harm'. Bowlby (1951; 1975; 1977) had intimated much concern about the separation of mothers from their infants although he considered attachment did not occur until about three months in the human species. This argument, too, could have contributed to the reasoning for what was perpetrated in hospitals as sound policy, in relation to early care giving and the neonate.

The physical condition of many mothers immediately after childbirth was not as good in earlier years as it is today. Along with social improvements and better general health, women are much more 'able' to interact and become involved in the caring of their infant now, compared to two decades ago.

☐ The pre-term infant

The pre-term infant and his mother provide observers with a unique opportunity to study the effects of maternal–child separation without the need to engineer distancing, as it is still the accepted norm to care for pre-term infants in a different environment from their mothers.

Children who are born pre-term are thought to be more at-risk of rejection, failure to thrive syndrome and non-accidental injury, than full-term infants (Gunter 1963). Observers have suggested that relationship differences exist between pre-term babies and their mothers and full-term infant/mother pairs. Mothers who are separated from their newborn pre-term infants may also experience later care-giving difficulties (Klaus & Kennell 1976). An earlier study by Leifer et al (1972) however, found no observed differences in maternal care-giving activities between three groups of mother-infant dyads having different separation experiences:

- Full-term babies (non-separated);

- Pre-term group (contact) parents encouraged to visit and handle their infants from day two;

- Pre-term group (separated) parents allowed only visual contact with babies during a three week period.

Although no differences were found in the quality of maternal care giving between the pre-term contact and separated groups it was noted that 'interaction' even in the contact group was low, the mothers visiting once only every six days to handle and feed their baby. At follow-up two years later though, other factors were considered and found to be different. Of the non-contact group (26) two mothers had relinquished custody of their infant and five mothers were divorced compared to one mother in the contact group (23).

A study by Minde et al (1978) compared the effects of high, medium and low levels of maternal stimulation of pre-term infants in a special care nursery in the USA. Mothers were observed visiting their infants soon after birth, during the mother's period of hospitalisation and after her discharge. The maternal-infant pairs were also observed at home one, two and three months after the baby's discharge from hospital nursery. Findings demonstrated that mothers who interacted consistently less with their infants soon after birth (low level stimulation) visited and telephoned the nursery less often than mothers who were observed to interact more with their infants at this time (high level stimulation). At follow up similar trends were demonstrated; low level stimulating mothers continued to interact less with their babies compared with the high level group. The mothers also reported poor relationships with their mothers and with the father of the baby. All, with the exception of one, had neither the support of a spouse nor friends in whom to confide at this time. The same authors report the reluctance of all mothers to touch their pre-term infant during the first two visits, despite being given verbal encouragement to do so, and advise that mothers of these babies may need to adjust to their infant's unexpected appearance by simply observing the neonate. The present policy, in some special care units, of offering detailed explanations about the baby's environment and monitoring equipment, in the absence of a request to do so, may interrupt the initial maternal-infant interaction at this time and work requires to be done to examine this. Minde *et al* (1978) suggest that a mother's early interaction with her pre-term infant may be a good indicator of her initial adjustment to the baby.

■ Neonatal abilities and the contribution to attachment

It is now quite clear that the newborn baby has a very great ability to learn. An expert on infant learning (Lipsitt 1965) has suggested that the newborn can learn better at this time than at any later age. The role of the midwife in her capacity as a teacher of parentcraft should endeavour to impart to mothers and fathers the known capabilities of their newborn baby, beginning as soon after birth as is appropriate to do so, and according to each parents' needs.

☐ Crying

Crying is considered to be the neonate's only means of communication. It occurs from the time of birth but it is some days or weeks before crying is accompanied by tears. Several distinct types of crying have been shown, representing hunger, pain or pleasure (Wasz-Hockert *et al* 1968; Wolff 1969). The mother's dilemma of learning to differentiate between her infant's crying types can be a most distressing experience, especially for the first time mother. It is suggested that midwifery personnel do not 'remove' the infant 'to settle him' but remain with the mother and allow her the benefit of learning the 'known' techniques which the midwife will use to soothe and settle the baby. It is surprising, for example, how many mothers do not hold the crying baby in an upright ventral position when attempting to comfort him until advised to do so. Korner and Thoman (1972) found that 80 per cent of their sample of crying infants cried less when they were put to the shoulder and held ventrally, compared to other common soothing procedures. The crying child is found to be more upsetting for some parents than for others and some mothers are more able to soothe and give comfort. Studies have demonstrated that crying can be increased by inappropriate rocking of the infant and also by inappropriate feeding (Smitherman 1969; Bell & Ainsworth 1972). It has also been noted that rooming-in mothers were able to interpret more information from their infant's cry than mothers who had experienced less contact with their baby at the same time (Greenberg *et al* 1973). For many abusing parents, crying seems to be by far the most upsetting behaviour in the child. It arouses intolerable anxiety and often results in injury to the child (Kempe & Kempe 1978). A crying infant usually elicits some form of response from the sensitive mother. Being able to determine the cause of crying and in turn managing successfully to soothe

the infant, is a rewarding experience for both mother and child and can add to the care giver's self esteem (Moss & Robson 1968).

☐ **Grasping**

Babies are born with the ability to finger-hold and this can be witnessed very soon after birth when mothers offer their forefinger to be grasped by the newborn. While most newly delivered mothers initiate finger-holding inter-action, observations would suggest that breast-feeding mothers in particular are more likely to continue with the practice during feeding than mothers who bottle feed. This author has also found that nursing mothers report synchrony between finger holding and continuous sucking phases, with relaxing of the hold by the infant during pauses in the sucking rhythm.

☐ **Rooting**

The rooting response is shown as a side to side movement of the infant's head in response to touching the baby anywhere near the mouth, and can be observed soon after birth. The response is an integral part of the feeding pattern and babies nuzzle towards the breast in anticipation whenever they are in the feeding position. Mothers who choose to bottle feed their infants occasionally express 'distaste' of the nuzzling action exhibited by their bottle-fed babies. By about the third month rooting is also elicited by the sight of the breast or bottle (Prechtl 1958).

☐ **Babkin's reflex**

When light pressure is applied to the palms of baby's hands, he will move his head and open his mouth in a demonstration of classical conditioning (Bower 1978).

☐ **Auditory/adult speech**

The uterus is not a sound proof chamber and it is believed that the fetus can hear sounds during his development. Ultrasound has been used to demon-strate babies' reactions *in utero* to 'engineered' noise like the dropping of a steel dish onto a hard floor. Pregnant women, too, are aware of changes in their fetus' pattern of movement when other fetal heart rates are being monitored electronically in the same ward or room, and the sound volume is pitched at a certain level.

Neonates respond to all sounds but most of all to speech and especially to the sound of their mother's voice. The infant's ability to differentiate between his mother's voice and others has been demonstrated in several ways using pupillary dilatation, smiling, visual attention and changes in behaviour as response indicators (Caldwell 1965; Banks & Wolfson 1967; Wahler 1967; Yarrow 1967; Fitzgerald 1968).

Adult speech to infants is characterised by higher and wider pitch ranges and is known as 'motherese'. Motherese has been widely reported cross culturally although its universality is disputed. A study by Farnald (1985) demonstrated that four month old infants had a significant preference for motherese speech as opposed to adult conversation type language. The high pitched human voice elicits the attention of the baby and is often demonstrated by women (and men) who raise the tone of their normal speaking voices to address the infant. When a neonate is held 'en face' at this time (at a distance of 8–10 inches pupil to pupil) he may appear to imitate the lip movements of the speaker.

The importance of the mother's speech to the child acquiring language in middle and working class families has been demonstrated by Dunn *et al* (1977). The group of mothers from working class families spent less time talking with their children about the books and pictures they were looking at compared to the group of mothers from middle class families. The middle class mothers also spent more time actively playing with their children and, even when busy with household tasks, were more likely to pay a great deal of attention to their child's activity. It is acknowledged that other differences between the two groups may contribute to the child's acquisition of language, including the mother–child relationship.

□ **Visual**

It is now known that babies from the time of birth are able to focus at a distance of 8–10 inches; any nearer or further away, the object of focus appears fuzzy (Schaffer 1971). The movements of the eyes are integrated with the movements of the head just as sucking is innately co-ordinated with rooting, swallowing and breathing (Schaffer 1971). Despite this knowledge, many people, including mothers and grandmothers, believe that babies are unable to 'see' until around 6 weeks of age. It is the duty of midwives to ensure that all mothers are informed of the true facts about the infant's visual abilities. It is also suggested that this information be given early and, where practical, demonstrated between a mother and her new baby. A moderate degree of photophobia has been noted during the early days of life and infants are more likely to open their eyes if the lighting around them is less harsh.

In observing mother–baby interactions, one is left in no doubt about the impact on the mother of eye to eye contact with her baby. Prince and Adams (1978) suggest that the care and attention the mother gives her baby is made much more rewarding by an attentive infant. Congenitally blind infants were described by Fraiberg (1974) who found that the absence of eye contact was a major problem which disrupted the mother's responsiveness towards the baby from birth onwards. The critical or sensitive period after birth, thought to be so important to the initiation of the mother–child relationship, may be for some the first time a mother consciously makes eye contact with her baby. Much more research requires to be done into whether early eye contact and verbal/non-verbal communication, after delivery, does affect the maternal–infant relationship and long term experiences of the child.

□ Olfactory perception

Neonates, at five days of age, can recognise the smell of their own mother's breast pads (McFarlane 1975). Should this ability be reciprocated in the mother it could probably be shown to have a bearing on the maternal/infant relationship. Several mothers indicate dislike of the odour of artificial milk as do some midwives when bottle feeding babies. Research would determine, among other factors, whether mothers who disliked the smell of the milk were less likely to cuddle their infant compared to those who did not find the milk smell 'unpleasant'.

□ Smiling

Mothers and midwives may believe that the newborn's smiles are caused by 'wind' although no evidence has been found to support this (Emde & Robinson 1976). The cursory smile of the newborn is nevertheless taken as a signal of the infant's pleasure and some mothers do ask whether the baby is really smiling. Smiling is of particular importance in the development of social interaction and babies do appear to pay more attention to the moving parts of the human face, that is, the eyes and the lips.

□ Touch

Apart from skin to skin contact between a mother and her infant soon after delivery, very little is written about touch and its effect on the infant. Observations suggest that the newborn uses his hands to explore different textures which surround him and he appears to prefer skin to other materials, although there is no research to support this theory. Unless an infant has been swaddled, he will choose to sleep, in most instances, with his hands in contact with his face. A baby will also 'caress' the skin of his mother's breast while nursing and although the effect of this is known on the mother, the question remains as to why the infant initiates such interaction. Further observations suggest that an infant's crying can be reduced during infliction of painful procedures such as heel pricking, when his mother is encouraged to remain with him and offer her forefingers to be grasped by the infant in both hands. Midwifery staff have been 'guilty' of encouraging mothers to 'disappear' while anything unpleasant was being done to their infant and this practice should probably be reconsidered in the interests of the mother–child relationship. To facilitate assessment of maternal care-giving using FIRST score (described on pages 78–9), infants were placed in bed with their mothers at 1–2 hours after birth (Salariya & Cater 1984). Modified skin contact was afforded mother and baby by placing the infant's naked feet upon the mother's unclothed thigh at this time. It was noted that when the mother moved, and her thigh became inaccessible to the infant, the baby extended one leg as far as was possible and was often seen to be making skin contact by only one big toe.

■ Parenting

Parenting has been described as 'the ability to recognise (with or without clear understanding) the needs of the child for:

● Physical care and protection;

● Nurturance;

● Love and the opportunity to relate to others;

● Bodily growth and the exercise of physical and mental function;

● Help in relating to the environment by way of organising and. mastering experience.

A parent must be able to meet these needs or at least facilitate their being met' (Kempe & Kempe 1978). Despite the importance attached to essential factors for parenting or care giving, it is estimated in some populations that one-third or more children grow up with parents or care-givers who do not provide such conditions (Bowlby 1977).

Some mothers have indicated that they did not love their baby at or around the time of birth and it may be presumed that this is not abnormal. It may be further believed that the 'unloved' neonate did successfully weather the storm until his mother's love was kindled. Babies are totally dependent for all their physical, emotional, mental and social needs on care givers who are normally their mothers, during the neonatal period. The majority of mothers would appear to express love, tenderness, concern and compassion at the outset while some mothers are less 'caring' of their infants at this time. Mother love is as essential to the child's mental health as vitamins and proteins are to his physical well being (Bowlby 1951). Love, according to Schaffer (1971), is an emotional involvement with another person which brings with it the capacity to experience a great range of feelings, from infinite tenderness to fierce possessiveness, from a willingness to sacrifice oneself for the sake of the other's well-being, to great surges of hostility and aggression.

Mothering was thought to be a natural instinct and the mother expressed this by cuddling and caressing her infant (Myles 1977). Oakley (1987) believes that 'a woman's relationship with her baby begins not only before birth but before conception. It has roots in her own babyhood, in the way she herself was mothered'.

Whether bonding, mothering or parenting is innate or learned, one cannot ignore official statistics about the number of children who do not appear to benefit from the 'natural instincts' of their mother. Theorists are agreed that the maternal/child relationship is a two way process and that infants may initiate some of the interaction at the earliest possible opportunity. Moss and Robson (1968) found that infants, given the opportunity, initiated 50 per cent or more of early interactions with the mother or care giver. Synchrony between adult speech sounds and infant body movement during periods of care-giving has been demonstrated as early as the first postnatal day, using special photographic techniques (Condon & Sander 1974).

In predicting successful and unsuccessful parenting, researchers found that information obtained during labour and post delivery observations resulted in 76.5 per cent correct predictions being made. They conclude that these assessments are very essential and that 'doctors and nurses, working with expectant mothers and parents during labour and post delivery, are ideally placed to make sensitive and significant observations of the way parents react to their new baby' (Grey et al 1977). Chappell and Sander (1979) recommend that the same mother-infant pair be observed several times before conclusions about their relationships were made and Macfarlane (1977) agrees that 'one off' observations of a mother interacting with her baby could be 'grossly misleading about her actual feelings'.

☐ **Bonding failure**

Researchers have described 'bonding failure' as the failure to develop normal parent–child love and suggest that if signs to this effect are recognised in the maternity unit, action can be taken to prevent abuse (Lynch & Roberts 1977). In a retrospective study, Lynch and Roberts compared the birth records of 50 children, referred because of actual or threatened abuse, with the birth records of another 50 (non-abused) children born at the same hospital. The researchers found five factors significantly more common in the abused group:

• Mother aged under 20 years at birth of first child;

• Evidence of maternal emotional disturbance;

• Referral of family to hospital social worker;

• Baby's admission to special care baby unit;

• Recorded concern over the mother's ability to care for her child.

Hospital staff had expressed direct concern in the records at the time of birth about the mother's 'ability' to cope with her child's physical or emotional needs; 'cannot stand her baby's cry', 'has not visited baby for more than a week', 'does not know how to respond to baby's needs' were typical written comments. The researchers examined all maternal records and found evidence of concern in 22 of the 'abused' group and only three in the control group. They advise that mothers who find difficulty in caring for their baby often give warning signals to maternity hospital staff although these do not necessarily lead to appropriate action being taken if and when they are reported.

Mothers who read their infant's cues correctly are more responsive to their cries, engage in more playful interaction and feed them on demand. Mothers at the other end of the scale tend to react less quickly (or not at all) to their infant's cries, spend more time giving physical care than in playful face-to-face interaction and tend to feed their baby at rigid regular intervals.

In a study by de Chateau *et al* (1978), left side preference for holding and carrying babies was demonstrated by 80 per cent of mothers, independent of handedness. The incidence of left side holding was lowered in mothers who had been separated from their infants immediately after birth. Non-separated, right holding mothers differed from left side holding ones in several ways; they held their babies with less body contact and perceived a delay in accepting the fetus or newborn as their own. At follow up, three years after delivery, the children had more frequent contact with Child Health Centres and the authors suggest that right side holding may, in some mothers, be an early sign of a disturbed mother-infant relationship.

☐ **Maltreatment**

Bowlby (1975) predicted that the attached infant would be strongly drawn to the attachment figure under conditions of stress, even if the attachment figure itself was the source of stress, but Lamb (1976) argues that attachment would not occur unless the social object behaved 'appropriately'.

Advocates of attachment theory suggest that many forms of psychiatric disturbance can be attributed to deviations in the development of attachment behaviour or to its failure (Bowlby 1977). When abused or neglected children of 18 months of age were observed with their biological or foster mothers, they demonstrated marked differences in the quality of adult-infant attachment (Lamb *et al* 1985). Maltreatment by mothers was associated with a marked increase in the number of children who experienced insecure relationships, even with foster mothers, but especially with the maltreating biological mothers. In contrast, maltreatment of the child by someone other than the biological mother appeared not to affect security of attachment between children and mother figures. The researchers note that much less attention has been paid to the effects of child abuse or neglect on children who have experienced the maltreatment during the earliest years of life.

Abused toddlers avoided both peers and care takers and were found to be more aggressive towards teachers than were non-abused children in a comparative study by George and Main (1979).

☐ **Child abuse**

It is suggested 'that abused children grow up to be abusing parents and the intervention and treatment we can offer serves not only to protect children now but helps to break the chain that binds future generations' (Kempe & Kempe 1978).

In a prospective study of 350 mothers, Grey *et al* (1977) examined many aspects of the mother, father and infant states, at or around the time of birth. Mothers completed a lengthy questionnaire, were interviewed and observed during labour and post delivery (by doctors and nurses) and at six weeks after the baby's birth. Some of the factors considered during the varying stages of the study are listed below because of their relevance as guidelines to holistic midwifery practice. These include:

- Parents' feelings towards the unborn child;

- Parents' living conditions if overcrowded;

- Amount of support and help to be expected from family or friends;

- Denial of the baby by the mother (for example, fostering a desire not to gain weight, refusing to talk about the situation and failing to make appropriate preparation for the baby);

- Feeling depressed and lonely about the pregnancy and delivery or experiencing other intolerable conditions of isolation or instability;

- Whether parents themselves had been neglected or abused;

- Lack of parental concern about the gender of the baby or his/her performance;

- Absence of a loving relationship between parents;

- Mothers who responded passively to their infant (did not hold, touch or examine them);

- Parents who reacted in a hostile manner towards their infant or made disparaging remarks about him/her;

- Mothers who avoided holding their baby 'en face' making eye contact impossible;

- Mothers who seemed to find their baby too demanding at feeding times or were repelled by the 'messiness' of it all;

- Mothers' distaste of having to change nappies;

- A mother's feeling of helplessness during her baby's crying periods;

- Partners who were jealous of their baby;

- Mothers who ignored or failed to respond to their baby's needs altogether and handed the responsibility over to doctors and nurses.

Starr (1982) found one of the few differences between abuse and control samples was that the abusing group saw child rearing as a simple rather than a complex task. In assessing maternal care giving ability during the early puerperium, using 'FIRST' score (see pages 78–9). Salariya and Cater (1984) noted that 'low scoring' mothers appeared to have little or no awareness of their poor care-giving capabilities and were very positive when asked 'how are you coping with your baby?' Invariably the reply was 'no problem' or 'OK'. This was in contrast to 'higher scoring' mothers who replied in less positive terms.

It is reported by Brown and Saqi (1988) that abusing parents have more negative conceptions of their children's behaviour than non-abusing parents and perceive their children to be more 'irritable and demanding'. The authors suggest that this may be related to the fact that abused children are more likely to have health problems, and eating or sleeping disturbances. An increase in child abuse amongst twins has been reported by Nelson and Martin (1985).

■ Recommendations for clinical practice in the light of currently available evidence

It has been suggested that the early management of a baby is a matter beyond conscious thought and deliberate intention. It is something that becomes possible only through love (Winnicott 1957). Medical and other sciences have made progress beyond belief yet many healthy babies, having survived the rigours of intrauterine development, labour and delivery, do not go on to enjoy a satisfactory quality of life.

Health is a state of complete physical, mental and social well being and not merely the absence of disease. Midwives have conscientiously adopted the medical model in the management of pregnancy, labour, delivery and postpartum. Their skills are updated to include new knowledge and many midwives extend their roles to effect repair of episiotomy wounds and to 'top up' epidural analgesia for example. Relatively little attention has been paid, however, to the importance of early mothering skills, considered by experts to be so essential to the short and long term experience of the child. The midwife's role in postpartum care is well known in relation to breast and bottle feeding, baby bathing and the reconstituting of milk formula, and each procedure is recorded in care plans and other 'nursing' notes accordingly. The recording of maternal care giving observations, if and when carried out, are not usually documented because the information is considered to be 'too sensitive'. Midwives, nevertheless, have made claim to being able to identify good, poor and indifferent maternal care giving and several researchers have recognised the contributions made by midwives in affecting this (Kempe & Kempe 1978; Lynch & Roberts 1977; Ounsted *et al* 1982). Because the information is considered to be 'too sensitive', verbal communication is often the favoured method by which reports of less than satisfactory care-giving are passed on from midwife to midwife.

Having recognised mothering impairment, midwives very often search for an excuse for the mother having behaved in this way and conclude, 'everything will be all right when mother and baby go home from hospital'. In believing this, midwives may be making irresponsible and even grave mistakes.

It is said that midwifery personnel are in the ideal position to monitor mother–child relationships 24 hours a day during the early puerperium, and no one would disagree with this. Controversy arises, however, as to *how* midwives should carry this out. Direct observation would appear to be the most reliable method of assessing mothering skills and the observer must have knowledge and ability to enable her to do this.

Child abuse and neglect both physical and emotional, are perpetrated by parents from all walks of life and therefore all mother–infant pairs should be 'screened' during the period of hospitalisation.

An assessment tool was designed to facilitate measurement of some aspects of maternal care-giving during the post partum period (Salariya & Cater 1984). The 'FIRST' score examines the mother's interest/ability in relation to her baby in respect of Feeding, Interest, Response, Speech (including eye contact) and Touch. The tool enables midwives to assess, implement and evaluate the mother's need for advice and support which may be required to enable the newly delivered mother to give holistic care to her infant. The recordings are scored numerically and the inter-observer reliability of the tool has been tested and proven.

Midwives have demonstrated that they can assess maternal care giving subjectively. Because personal feelings are 'difficult' to record, many opinions about care-giving are lost and this is most regrettable. No other professional is in a more privileged position to identify maternal/child relationships at their very initiation and the midwife must appreciate this responsibility. To make objective assessment of early relationships using appropriate tools would enable midwives to standardise such observations. The value of early assessments would soon be known. Community midwives, health visitors, social workers, paediatricians and psychologists could validate the worth of such communication as the first link in a chain of screening procedures to identify children at risk. In the words of Kempe and Kempe (1978), 'To provide excellent obstetric, postnatal and paediatric care in our hospitals makes very little sense if we fail to observe initial relationships between parents and their neonate, at this time'.

■ Practice check

Try to use every opportunity to observe (unobtrusively) mothers, fathers and babies interacting.

- During the course of 24 hours, how often are babies 'disturbed' to allow routine examination or handling by midwives, by paediatricians, by technicians, by the photographer, by visitors and by others?
- Observe how many mothers (and midwives) display left-side preference holding of infants as opposed to right-side holding.
- During bottle feeding, observe how infants are held by mothers (and midwives). Is the position and distance (eye to eye) similar to that used for breastfeeding?
- Do all mothers in your care know the visual abilities of their newborn baby?
- Are mothers encouraged to be present with their baby at times of physical examination and/or during other invasive procedures?
- You are asked by a mother, 'what is meant by mother–infant attachment?' How would you reply?.

■ References

Ainsworth M D 1962 The effects of maternal deprivation: a review of findings and controversy in the context of research strategy. In Deprivation of maternal care: 62. WHO, Geneva

Ainsworth M D S, Bell S M 1970 Attachment by the behaviour of one year olds in a strange situation. Child Development 41: 49–67

Anisfeld E, Lipper E 1983 Early contact, social support and mother-infant bonding. Pediatrics 72: 79–83

Banks J H, Wolfson J H 1967 Differential cardiac response of infants to mother and stranger. Paper to the Eastern Psychological Association, Philadelphia, cited by Schaffer (1971), page 86

Bell S M, Ainsworth M D S 1972 Infant crying and maternal responsiveness. Child Development 43: 1171–90

Bower S M, Miller B C 1980 Parental attachment behaviour as related to presence at delivery and parenthood classes. Nursing Research 29: 307–11

Bower T G R 1978 The world of the newborn. In Human development. Freeman, San Francisco

Bowlby J 1951 Maternal care and mental health. A Report by E J M Bowlby. WHO, Geneva

Bowlby J 1969 Attachment and loss, Vol 1 Attachment. Hogarth Press, London

Bowlby J 1975 Attachment and loss, Vol 2 Separation, anxiety and anger. Penguin Books, Harmondsworth

Bowlby J 1977 The making and breaking of affectional bonds. British Journal of Psychiatry 130: 201–10

Boyd S T 1981 Parent education: paternal involvement in the behaviour assessment of the newborn. Paper presented at the Conference of the Association for the Care of Children's Health, Toronto, May 1981

Browne K, Saqi S 1988 Early prediction and prevention of child abuse. Browne K, Davies C and Stratton P (eds), John Wiley and Sons Ltd, Chichester

Caldwell B M 1965 Visual and emotional reactions of an infant to his mother and other adult females. Paper to the Tavistock Study Group on Mother–Infant Interaction, London, cited by Schaffer (1971), page 88

Campbell S B G, Taylor P M 1980 Bonding and theoretical issues. In Taylor, PM (ed) Parent-infant relationships. Grune & Stratton, New York

Chappell P, Sander L W 1979 Mutual regulation of the neonatal-maternal interactive process: context for the origins of communication. In Bullowa M (ed) Before speech: the beginning of interpersonal communication. Cambridge University Press, Cambridge

Condon W, Sander L 1974 Synchronization of neonate movement with adult speech: interactional participation and language acquisition. Science 183: 99–101

de Chateau P, Wiberg B 1977 Long-term effect on mother-infant behaviour of extra contact during the first hour post partum II. A follow-up at three months. Acta Paediatrica Scandinavica 66: 145–51

de Chateau P, Holmberg H, Winberg J 1978 Left side preference in holding and carrying newborn infants. Acta Paediatrica Scandinavica 67: 169–75

Dunn J, Wooding C, Hermann J 1977 Mothers' speech to young children: variation in context. Developmental Medicine and Child Neurology 19: 629–38

Emde R N, Robinson J 1976 The first two months: recent research in developmental psychobiology and the changing view of the newborn. In Noshpitz J, Call J (eds) Basic handbook of child psychiatry. Basic Books, New York

Farnald A 1985 Four month old infants prefer to listen to motherese. Infant
    Behaviour and Development   8: 181–95
Fitzgerald H E 1968 Autonomic pupillary reflex activity during early infancy, and
    its relation to social and non-social visual stimuli. Journal of Experimental
    Child Psychology   5: 171–84
Fraiberg S 1974 Blind infants and their mothers. In Lewis M, Rosenblum L (eds)
    The effects of the infant on its caregiver: 215–33. John Wiley, New York
George C, Main M 1979 Social interactions of young abused children: approach,
    avoidance and aggression. Child Development   50: 306–18
Goldberg S 1983 Parent infant bonding: another look. Child Development   54:
    1355–82
Grey J, Cutler C, Dean J, Kempe H 1977 Prediction and prevention of child
    abuse and neglect. Child Abuse and Neglect   1 (1): 45–58
Greenberg D J, O'Donnell W J, Crawford D 1973 Complexity levels, habituation
    and individual differences in early infancy. Child Development   44: 469–74
Greenberg N, Morris N 1974 Engrossment: the newborn's impact upon the
    father. American Journal of Orthopsychiatry   4: 520–31
Gunter L M 1963 Psychopathology and stress in the life experience of mothers of
    premature infants. American Journal of Obstetrics and Gynecology   86: 333
Hales D J, Lozoff B, Sosa R, Kennell J H 1977 Defining the limits of the
    maternal sensitive period. Developmental Medicine and Child Neurology
    19: 454–61
Hess E H 1973 Imprinting. Van Nostrand, New York
Keller W D, Hildebrandt K A, Richards M E 1985 Effects of extended
    father-infant contact during the newborn period. Infant behaviour and
    development   8: 337–50
Kempe R S, Kempe C H 1978 The abusive parent. In Bruner J, Cole M, Lloyd B
    (eds) Child abuse. Fontana/Open Books Original, London
Kennell J H, Trause M A, Klaus M H 1975 Evidence for a sensitive period in the
    human mother. In CIBA Foundation Symposium 33: Parent–infant
    interaction. Elsevier, Amsterdam
Klaus M H, Jerauld R, Kreger N C, McAlpine W, Steffa M, Kennell J H 1972
    Maternal attachment: importance of the first post-partum days. New England
    Journal of Medicine   286: 460–63
Klaus M H, Kennell J H 1976 Maternal infant bonding. Mosby, St Louis
Korner A, Thoman E 1972 The relative efficacy of contact and vestibular
    proprioceptive stimulation in soothing neonates. Child Development   43:
    443–53
Lamb M E 1976 The role of the father in child development. John Wiley, New
    York
Lamb M E, Gaensbauer T J, Malkin C M, Schultz L A 1985 The effects of child
    maltreatment on security of infant–adult attachment. Infant Behaviour and
    Development   8: 35–45
Leifer A D, Leiderman P H, Barnett C R, Williams J A 1972 Effects of mother–
    infant separation on maternal attachment behaviour. Child Development
    43: 1203–18
Lipsitt L P 1965 Learning in the human infant. In Stevenson H W, Rheingold H
    L, Hess E (eds) Early behaviour: comparative and developmental approaches.
    John Wiley, New York

Liptak G S, Keller B B, Feldman A W, Chamberlin R W 1983 Enhancing infant development and parent–practitioner interaction with the Brazelton neonatal assessment scale. Pediatrics 72: 71–8

Lynch M A, Roberts J 1977 Predicting child abuse: signs of bonding failure in the maternity hospital. British Medical Journal 1: 624–26

McFarlane A 1975 Olfaction in the development of social preferences in the human neonate. In CIBA Foundation Symposium 33: Parent–infant interaction. Elsevier, Amsterdam

Macfarlane A 1977 The psychology of childbirth. Fontana, London

Minde K, Trehub S, Corter C, Boukydis C, Celhoffer L, Marton P 1978 Mother–child relationships on the premature nursery: an observational study. Pediatrics 61: 373–79

Moss H A, Robson K 1968 Early social visual behaviour. Child Development 39: 401–08

Myles, M 1977 Myles textbook for midwives, 8th ed: 448. Churchill Livingstone, Edinburgh

Nelson H B, Martin C A 1985 Increased child abuse in twins. Child Abuse and Neglect 9 (4): 501–05

Oakley A 1987 Mother love – do midwives help or hinder? Lancet i: 379

Ounsted C, Roberts J C, Gordon M, Milligan B 1982 Fourth goal of perinatal medicine. British Medical Journal 284: 879–82

Parke R, O'Leary S E 1976 Family interaction in the newborn period: some findings, some observations and some unresolved issues. In Meacham J, Riegel K (eds) Developing individual in a changing world. Mouton, The Hague

Prechtl H F R 1958 The directed head turning response and allied movements of the human baby. Behaviour 13: 212–42

Prince J, Adams M E 1978 Minds, mothers and midwives: the psychology of childbirth. Churchill Livingstone, Edinburgh

Robson E M, Powell E 1982 Early maternal attachments. In Brockington I F, Kumar R (eds) Mothering and mental illness. Academic Press, London

Salariya E M, Cater J I 1984 Mother–child relationship – FIRST score. Journal of Advanced Nursing 9: 589–95

Schaffer H R 1971 The growth of sociability. Penguin Books, Harmondsworth

Schaffer H R, Emerson P E 1964 The development of social attachments in infancy. Monographs of the Society for Research in Child Development 29 (3): 3–76

Schaffer R 1982 Love, hate and indifference. In Bruner J, Cole M, Lloyd B (eds) Mothering: the developing child. Fontana/Open Books Original, London

Smitherman C 1989 The vocal behaviour of infants as related to the nursing procedure of rocking. Nursing Research 18: 256–58

Starr R H Jr 1982 A research based approach to the prediction of child abuse. In Child abuse and prediction: policy implications. Ballinger, Cambridge, Mass

Wahler R G 1967 Infant social attachments: a reinforcement theory interpretation and investigation. Child Development 38: 1079–88

Wasz-Hockert O, Lind J, Vuorenkoski V, Partanen T, Valanne E 1968 The infant cry, a spectrographic and auditory analysis. Spastics International Medical Publications/Heinemann, London

Winnicott D W 1957 The child and the outside world. Tavistock Publications, London

Winnicott D W 1968 The child, the family, and the outside world. Penguin Books, Harmondsworth

Wolff P H 1969 The natural history of crying and other vocalizations in early infancy. In Foss B M (ed) Determinants of infant behaviour IV. Methuen, London

Yarrow L J 1967 The development of focused relationships during infancy. In Hellmuth J (ed) Exceptional infant, Vol 1. Seattle Special Child Publications, Seattle

■ Suggested further reading

Dick D 1987 Yesterday's babies. The Bodley Head, London

Kempe R S, Kempe C H 1978 The abusive parent. In Bruner J, Cole M, Lloyd B (eds) Child abuse. Fontana/Open Books Original, London

Mullan B 1979 Are mothers really necessary? Boxtree, London

Pearce J C 1979 Magical child. Paladin, Granada, London

Schaffer R 1982 Love, hate and indifference. In Bruner J, Cole M, Lloyd B (eds) Mothering: the developing child, 4th impression. Fontana/Open Books Original, London

Chapter 5

Care of the umbilical cord

Janet Rush

While performing a vital role for survival of the fetus, after delivery the umbilical cord stump is a redundant feature of the term newborn. It does, however, receive attention and activity by maternity staff and concern by parents. As it is the only open area of the baby's body, potentially problems can develop. In most societies there are routines for the care of the cord to facilitate drying and separation, and to prevent bacterial colonisation and infection, or cross-infection to others. Care of the cord is not a new concept and procedures for tying and wrapping it, followed by abdominal binding, have been meticulously described (Barrett 1851). Similarly, applications of chemicals to the cord are neither recent innovations nor simply responses to twentieth century medicine alone (Brown 1932).

Early postpartum care in Europe and North America occurs mostly in hospitals and care has typically been identified with sick bed protocols, rigid regimens and surgical wards. Fear of overwhelming infection in the nursery and staphylococcal epidemics justified compliance with routine procedures. Care was assumed only by nurses, midwives or doctors, and infants were separated into nurseries regulated by strict rules for infection control such as medicated bathing, visiting restrictions, caregiver apparel, inspection, nappy changing and cord treatments.

Trends in the 1950s and 1960s contributed to a growing dissatisfaction with the rigid hospital approach (Rush et al 1989). A new consumerism emerged and concepts such as family centred maternity care, attachment and rooming-in provided an alternative to usual practice. Parallel changes in a decreased length of stay and in the teaching and advocacy roles of the nurse/midwife supported the trends for more flexibility in obstetric units. While satisfaction was a strongly valued outcome for care, safety, especially concerning infection control for the newborn, continued to direct practice. Successful healing of the umbilical cord is one desired outcome related to the safety portion of the equation. It is generally felt that effective care (inspection, treatment, parent teaching and reporting) will prevent or detect the trauma or infection that can negatively affect the health of the newborn.

This chapter will provide a background against which to understand the importance of cord care in the term neonate. Reports of controlled trials will be discussed with recommendations for further research including the presentation of a design with which to evaluate practice in any setting.

■ It is assumed that you are already aware of the following:

- The structure of the fetal circulation and how it works;
- The anatomy of the umbilical cord;
- Changes in newborn circulation following delivery relative to the umbilical cord;
- The normal length of time taken for cord separation and the reasons for its occurrence;
- The principles of bacterial colonisation in the newborn;
- The significance of *Staphylococcus aureus* as a nosocomial pathogen;
- The importance of the caregiver's hands in the transmission of bacteria;
- The difference between colonisation and infection;
- The infection prevention strategies and cord treatments currently in use in your unit.

■ The epidemiological triangle – 'host', 'environment' and 'agent'

The fact that newborns may become colonised with a pathogen while in the hospital implies a dynamic relationship. The epidemiological triangle (Fig. 5.1) provides a useful framework for background information.

The newborn is a special 'host', described as susceptible to infection with no protective flora at birth (American Academy of Pediatrics 1974). Normal skin flora begin to be acquired within 24 hours. The flora reflect the environment and the maternal flora, and potentially harmful species are seldom found (Davies 1971; Hurwitz 1981). The newborn's skin has a lower pH than that of the adult, due to scanty sweat and sebaceous secretions, and this acid mantle acts as a natural bacterial inhibitor (Stroud 1982). The baby is born with a natural break in the skin, like a wound, that is the umbilicus. This affords an opportunity for bacterial colonisation and, in some instances, infection.

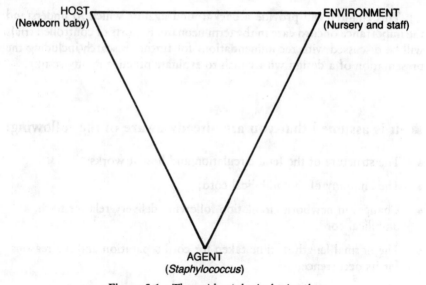

Figure 5.1 The epidemiological triangle

The umbilical stump is approximately 2–5 centimetres in length, following clamping and cutting at delivery. The external remnants of a vein and two arteries within the Wharton's jelly and surrounded by epithelial cells are no longer supplied with nourishment. Drying, atrophy and thrombosis starts immediately and when complete, the dark, hardened stump separates. This may take from 5–15 days (Wilson *et al* 1985). The mechanics of cord separation are not completely known (Schuman & Oksol 1985), but it is during this process that the cord can be colonised with bacteria, especially *staphylococcus* (*S.*) *aureus*. The umbilicus is one of the first sites for *S. aureus* colonisation (Gezon *et al* 1973). Once colonised, the infant has a potential for local or systemic infection and acts as a reservoir of bacteria capable of causing cross-infection in the maternity ward. Accumulated urine or stool within the nappy (in some settings a plastic covered disposable product) can favour bacterial growth close to the umbilical site or come in contact with the folds of tissue at the base of the cord stump. Frequent handling at nappy changes exposes the area to the hands of caregivers. Newborn boys, if circumcised, are also subjected to increased handling around the area of the cord.

The most troublesome 'agent' in normal nurseries is *S. aureus*, a gram positive cocci, an aerobe or facultative anaerobe. It grows best between 5–46°C and favours high concentrations of sodium chloride (Youmans *et al* 1975). Although many other antigens (Group B *Streptococci*; the HIV, hepatitis B and herpes viruses) are responsible for newborn morbidity (Larson 1987), it is *S. aureus* which is hospital-acquired and the frequent causative agent in nursery epidemics. The organism is carried in the anterior nares of health care personnel. The carriage rate among staff has been reported between 20–75 per cent (Youmans *et al* 1975; Smith 1979), as opposed to 5 per cent in the general population. While transmission of *S. aureus* by air, dust and fomites occurs, the hands are the most important carriers. Because nasal flora are found on the hands, and hands can colonise or become colonised by infants, the personnel's role in transmission of the agent is of the utmost importance.

The 'environment' consists of the external conditions and influences affecting the life and development of the organism (Murray & Zentner 1975). Notwithstanding the susceptibility of the baby, hospital settings are notorious bacterial reservoirs. Newborns are handled frequently by many professionals (a group which is known to have high carriage rates of *S. aureus*). Nursing, housekeeping and hospital policies for hand washing, apparel, assignment of duties, dust control, visitors, length of stay, supplies, equipment and skin and cord care have had long histories. Routine surveillance of the colonisation rate (the percentage of infants assessed via microbiological culture to have the presence of bacteria without clinical disease), has been widely used to measure the effectiveness of existing maternity infection control policies or of the introduction of new routines. It is debatable whether colonisation predicts overt newborn disease (Wang *et al* 1987). It is generally felt, however, that higher than normal rates (25–50 per cent) could predict a nursery epidemic (Harris & Polin 1983; Bennett & Brachman 1986) and hospitals adopt practices that keep the rates low.

Preventing or treating umbilical cord colonisation has been attempted through the use of various practices and chemical agents, mostly infant bathing and topical applications of powders, ointments, alcohol or other preparations. While trials of routine bathing with special additives (mostly hexachlorophene) were shown to reduce high nursery colonisation rates, reports of umbilical cord treatments demonstrated greater effectiveness (Rush *et al* 1989).

■ **A critical appraisal of the research**

In the first controlled trial of 'triple dye' (brilliant green, proflavin, hemisulphate and crystal violet in aqueous solution) to the cord stump, Jellard (1957) showed that *S. aureus* colonisation of the skin could be reduced and this effect was confirmed by others over the subsequent three decades (see Table 5.1). These controlled trials have not provided adequate information about the effect of the treatment on overt infection, but they do demonstrate a significant reduction in colonisation, a clinically acceptable outcome to most.

Of the various methods used to treat the umbilical cord, only neomycin has been shown to reduce the colonisation rate more effectively than triple

Table 5.1 Effect of triple dye on colonisation rate of *Staphylococcus aureus*

Study	Date	Experimental (Triple dye)		Control	
		n	%	n	%
Jellard	1957	10/50	20.0	26/49	53.0
Pildes *et al*	1973	56/531	10.5	148/207	71.5
Coyer	1975	110/270	40.7	36/52	69.2
Speck *et al*	1977	17/62	27.4	25/63	39.7
Barrett *et al*	1979	15/100	15.0	72/100	72.0
Gladstone *et al*	1988	0/48	0	35/87	40.0

dye. This was reported by Coyer (1975) where the neomycin cohort (271 in number) experienced a *S. aureus* colonisation rate of 27.3 per cent versus the triple dye group (of 270 babies) where a rate of 40 per cent was observed. The effects of silver sulphadiazine versus triple dye have been reported in four trials (see Table 5.2). In each it was concluded that triple dye was more effective in reducing the incidence of umbilical cord colonisation at 48 hours.

Other preparations currently in use, as well as the practice of no treatment or water cleansing, have not been adequately evaluated and/or compared to the triple dye standard. These practices relate to commercial interests, habit or there being no observable problem or financial burden to have stimulated rigorous scientific evaluation. The wide variety in Europe and North America suggests an uncertainty about what is most effective. A survey of 1,200 American hospitals (Martin *et al* 1983) cites the use of isopropyl alcohol as the most widely used agent (40 per cent), followed by triple dye (38 per cent), a combination of the two (14 per cent), bacitracin

Table 5.2 Effect of silver sulphadiazine versus triple dye on umbilical colonisation

Study	Date	Experimental (Silver sulphadiazine)		Control (Triple dye)	
		n	%	n	%
Speck *et al*	1977	31/89	34.8	25/89	28.1
Barrett *et al*	1979	81/100	81.0	55/100	55.0
Speck *et al*	1980	38/82	46.3	12/80	15.0
Gladstone *et al*	1988	4/42	10.0	0/14	0

(5 per cent) and iodophor (3 per cent). Other reports describe the use of chlorhexidine (Meberg & Schøyen 1985), various soaps (Coyer 1974; Barrett *et al* 1979; Martin *et al* 1983; Meberg & Schøyen 1985), neosporin (Coyer 1975), bismuth (Arad *et al* 1981) and ethyl alcohol (this author's personal experience).

Hospital infection outcomes are seldom reported in the controlled trials, however, the available evidence shows that there is no difference when silver sulphadiazine is compared to triple dye (Speck *et al* 1977), when triple dye, proviodine and silver sulphadiazine are compared (Gladstone *et al* 1988), or when triple dye is compared to alcohol (Schuman & Oksol 1985).

Earlier separation of the cord obviates the need for prolonged treatment, attention and concern by parents or nurse/midwives. Should no difference in clinical outcomes be observed between the various practices, then separation time and parent satisfaction are the next most important considerations.

The studies (see Table 5.3) reveal that the choice of cord treatment affects the rate at which the cord stump heals (Alder *et al* 1980; Arad *et al* 1981; Lawrence 1982; Barr 1984; Schuman & Oksol 1985; Wilson *et al* 1985; Mugford *et al* 1986; Gladstone *et al* 1988; Salariya & Kowbus 1988).

A longer number of days to separation is consistently observed with triple dye treatment (12–17 days). This was observed in case series data (Wilson *et al* 1985) and in controlled trials comparing it to alcohol (Schuman & Oksol 1985) and to other agents (Gladstone *et al* 1988). Only one report (Arad *et al* 1981) describes triple dye as causing shorter separation time than other agents.

Because powders, alcohol, water cleansing and no treatment were shown to promote more rapid drying and healing (with no observable concerns about infection), there is scope for large trials comparing colonisation, infection, separation and economic considerations among the interventions.

■ Recommendations for clinical practice

There is no solid, scientific basis for selecting from the variety of measures used to treat the cord because the trials have not been large enough to distinguish differences in infection rates. Based on the evidence of the research with the strongest designs (the controlled trials) triple dye is an effective prophylactic for routine use. Neomycin powder is an effective but more expensive alternative. There is no sound evidence as yet to justify the use of the various other agents. Dry care or no treatment (beyond general cleanliness) has also not been adequately tested. Consistent in all discussions

Table 5.3 Umbilical cord mean separation time

Study	Design	Treatment	n	Separation time (days)
Alder et al (1980)	Random selection (2 wards)	1% Chlorhexidine powder and 3% zince oxide	87	6.0
		0.33% hexachlorophene powder and 3% zinc oxide	87	6.0
Arad et al (1981)	RCT	Triple dye	36	7.7
		1% neomycin	26	12.0
		1% silver sulphadiazine	25	10.6
		Bismuth subgallate	34	6.4
Lawrence (1982)	2 ward comparison	0.33% hexachlorophene powder	100	6.6
		Alcohol swab and powder	100	7.1
Barr (1984)	Survey (2 hospitals)	Alcohol swab and cicatrin prn	83	8.1
		Water cleansing	34	6.2
Schuman & Oksol (1985)	RCT	Triple dye	35	15.7
		Isopropyl alcohol	36	10.7
Wilson et al (1985)	Survey	Triple dye	240	15.0
*Mugford et al (1986)	RCT	Zinc powder	199	6.3
		0.33% hexachlorophene powder	202	6.9
		Zinc oxide and alum	197	7.2
		No powder	202	8.1
Salariya & Kowbus (1988)	4 ward comparison	No treatment	100	7.1
		Alcohol swab and 0.33% hexachlorophene powder	100	7.1
		Alcohol swab	100	7.9
		0.33% hexachlorophene powder	100	6.6
Gladstone et al (1988)	RCT	Triple dye (daily)	14	17.4
		Triple dye (once) and alcohol (daily)	53	12.5
		Triple dye (once)	48	12.9
		Proviodine (daily)	48	9.9
		Silver sulphadiazine (daily)	44	13.8
		Bacitracin ointment (daily)	42	11.8

* Treatments were combined with various cleansing and frequency factors

of maternity infection control is the importance of hand washing. While it is clearly not ethical to evaluate the effect of this action, it would be of interest to compare care by different hands, that is cord care by the nurse/midwife versus cord care by the mother.

☐ **The role of the nurse/midwife involves:**

- Initial assessment (two arteries, one vein, clamp secure, no oozing, maternal and delivery histories for potential infection);
- Early observation (for atrophy and signs of infection);
- Measures to prevent cross-contamination (meticulous hand washing, rooming-in, individual infant items);
- Skin/cord care (avoiding cord irritation from clothing, cleansing of cord if soiled at nappy change, avoiding using fingers for application of cord treatment, avoiding the use of lotions near the cord);
- Reporting unusual signs;
- Providing teaching and practice time for parents.

Teaching parents the nature of cord separation, ongoing assessment and general care is an integral part of postpartum care. In Britain, midwives are required to provide visits until the umbilical stump is separated and healed (Mugford *et al* 1986). This is not the follow-up routine in North America. Parents provided with information, who demonstrate the required skill and knowledge, can be discharged home with little need for continued professional observations. It is the experience of this author that parents can cope with the expectations related to cord care and will report unusual problems. The health care provider can then attend to the reinforcement of the parent role rather than assuming it.

☐ **The effectiveness of bathing**

Recommendations (American Academy of Pediatrics 1974; Health and Welfare Canada 1987; American Academy of Pediatrics and the American College of Obstetricians and Gynecologists 1988) direct that babies should not be bathed routinely. Even so, survey data indicates that 93 per cent of hospitals continue this practice (Martin *et al* 1983). Daily baths, in most North American nurseries, are sponge baths ('topping and tailing') and mothers, over the years, have been advised not to use an infant bathtub until the cord has separated. It has been assumed that immersing the cord in water may promote infection or prevent drying, delaying separation.

A randomised controlled trial (Rush 1986) to evaluate the effectiveness of daily bathing versus no bathing or dry skin care, found no statistically significant difference in umbilical cord *S. aureus* colonisation rates between groups. In this study, following an initial bath, normal newborns were randomly allocated to a study group where they were sponged only if soiled or to a control group where the babies had a daily bath in an infant bathtub. Mild, nonmedicated soap was used for the bath. It was concluded that routine bathing is not a determinant in colonisation and that immersing the newborn in a tub is not a harmful intervention. Practice changes occurred to support the view that bathing should not be considered an infection control measure but rather an excellent time for teaching, parent contact, practice and building confidence.

Decisions about the effectiveness of the current cord care regimen in any setting are best undertaken using a strong experimental design. The most rigorous is the randomised controlled trial where newborns are placed randomly into one of two or more groups and followed up for a defined period of time to observe the outcome(s) of choice. Figure 5.2 offers such a design for consideration.

Consecutive admissions to the unit should be used and only those eligible be included in the study. In a study of term newborns include those of 37 weeks gestation or more, those with an Apgar score of at least 7 at five minutes, those not clinically ill or who have not spent a period of time in a special care unit. This assures like subjects at the outset. Written consent from parents is not only ethically essential but their co-operation is valuable in keeping the procedure for each group as pure as possible. The number of subjects required is a mathematical manoeuvre and the assistance of a statistician is invaluable. The figure required must be sufficient to demonstrate that any difference in outcome is related to the experimental manoeuvre, rather than chance or coincidence.

Demographic variables about the baby, the mother and the delivery that may possibly affect outcome should be collected and reported. Environmental factors are also important to describe as they help to compare settings, generalise results or ask new questions. Therefore, data should be documented about previous colonisation rates, time of year, staff nasal carriage rate, length of stay, rooming-in, general care, number of staff, visiting, ward census (occupancy rates), those subjects ineligible or refusing and the definition of the outcome.

Randomising to the experimental or control group(s) must take place as a blind event thereby strengthening the likelihood of the variables being equally distributed among the groups. Random number tables from computer programmes or statistics texts can be used to allocate the subjects, and opaque envelopes containing the choice of treatment for each consecutive baby assures objectivity. The protocol for each group must be strictly adhered to by staff and/or parents (or the subject identified). Blindness as to which subject is receiving which intervention is ideal. Where this is not

THE QUESTION

IS UMBILICAL CORD TREATMENT EFFECTIVE, COMPARED TO
THE CONTROL GROUP, IN PRODUCING THE DESIRED OUTCOME?

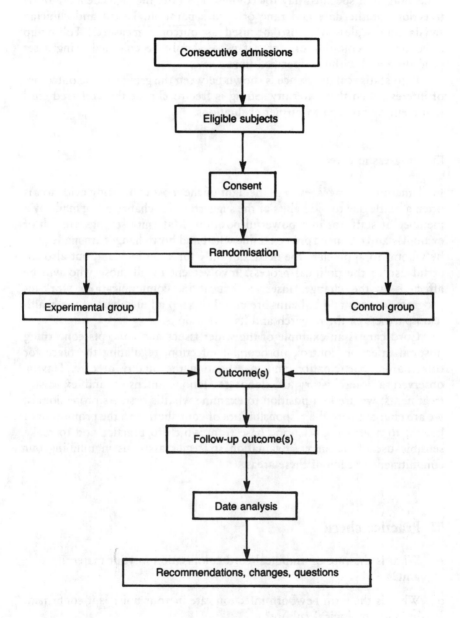

Figure 5.2   Randomised controlled design

possible (due to skin tinting or obvious differences in agents or frequencies), audits of the procedures or evaluators who are blind to the subjects' groups are adequate.

The outcome procedures must also be strictly followed whether it be the collection on a specified day for colonisation rate, the signs defining overt infection, or the date and time of cord separation. Parent and clinician satisfaction scales may also be used as outcome measures. Follow-up infection and colonisation data, if used, should be collected using a set procedure and within a specified time.

If no statistical difference is shown between the groups in the outcomes of interest, then the maternity setting is free to choose the preferred cord treatment or proceed to further evaluations.

☐ **Progress in care**

Implementing changes, even in the light of the most convincing evidence, is often a battle due to old habits or the suggestion for change being made by a member of staff not in a powerful position. Maternity settings are full of examples and one need only examine when and how changes are made (and by whom) to appreciate the need, not only for scientific data, but also for artful use of the political process. Involvement of all those who will be affected by the change, inservice education, communication, work-in-progress sessions and bulletins are useful to keep all members of the health team partners in the research and its conclusions.

Cord care is an example of the wider issues and concepts concerning hospital infection control, nosocomial infection, regulating the place for care, parent participation and investigating the quality of care. Having observed a long history of elaborate, labour intensive and expensive treatments, we are in a position to examine what is best. As professionals, we are charged with the responsibilities of contributing to the promotion of health, to a growing scientific base from which to practice and to make sensible use of resources. Evaluation strategies assist us in fulfilling our commitment in each of these areas.

■ **Practice check**

● What is the rate of umbilical cord colonisation in your maternity unit?

● What is the term newborn infection rate in your unit? Is it confirmed by microbiological culture?

● Is there a procedure for care that is practised in the same way by all?

- Can one assess, via the clinical record, that the cord area has been observed on a daily basis? Are the descriptors measurable and understood by all clinicians?

- Is hand washing before infant contact monitored?

- Can sound rationale be articulated for any other infection control routine – for example, limiting visiting by siblings, special apparel for handling babies, use of antiseptic agents, rooming-in, single or unit dose items, eye prophylaxis, length of hospital stay?

- What resources are available to conduct a research project to evaluate the effectiveness of your cord care routines?

- What instruction is given to mothers/fathers about care of the cord? Do they know the signs and symptoms of problems? Is the information reinforced by handout literature or follow-up? Are they given an opportunity to practice with the encouragement of the hospital staff?

- Is there, in your setting, the potential for cross-infection due to communal use of items? Can items for infant care be individual and contained with the cot?

- Are maternity infection control practices (by midwives, housekeepers, doctors and the administration) documented and reviewed regularly?

- Is there an infection control committee or officer?

- How are policies or procedures made, changed or reviewed in your setting?

■ References

Alder V G, Burman D, Simpson R A, Fysh J, Gillespie W A 1980 Comparison of hexachlorophene and chlorhexidane powders in prevention of neonatal infection. Archives of Disease in Childhood 55: 277–80

American Academy of Pediatrics, Committee on the Fetus and Newborn 1974 Skin care of the newborn. Pediatrics 54 (6): 682–83

American Academy of Pediatrics and the American College of Obstetricians and Gynaecologists 1988 Guidelines for perinatal care. Washington DC

Arad H, Eyal F, Farnmesser P 1981 Umbilical care and cord separation. Archives of Disease in Childhood 56: 887–88

Barr J 1984 The umbilical cord: to treat or not to treat? Midwives Chronicle 97 (1159): 224–26

Barrett F F, Mason E O, Fleming D 1979 The effects of three core care regimes on bacterial colonization of normal newborn infants. Journal of Pediatrics 94 (5): 796–800

Barrett T 1851 Advice on the management of children in early infancy. Binns and Goodwin, Bath

Bennett J V, Brachman P S 1986 Hospital infections (2nd edn): 490–1. Little Brown & Co, Boston, Toronto

Brown A 1932 The normal child: its care and feeding (3rd edn) McClelland and Stewart, Toronto

Coyer W F 1974 Phisohex versus topical gentamycin in the clinical control of *Staphylococcus aureus* colonization. Pediatric Research   8 (423): 149

Coyer W F 1975 Neonatal skin care and the prevention of *Staphylococcus aureus* colonization. Pediatric Research   9: 339

Davies P A 1971 Bacterial infections in the fetus and newborn. Archives of Disease in Childhood   46: 1–27

Gezon H M, Thompson D J, Rogers K D, Hatch T F, Rycheck R R, Yee R B 1973 Control of staphylococcal infections and disease in the newborn through the use of hexachlorophene. Pediatrics   51 (2): 331–43

Gladstone I M, Clapper I, Thorpe J W, Wright D I 1988 Randomized study of six cord care regimes. Clinical Pediatrics   27 (3): 127–29

Harris M C, Polin R A 1983 Neonatal septicemia. Pediatric Clinics of North America   30 (2): 243–58

Health and Welfare Canada 1987 Family-centred maternity and newborn care. National Guidelines, Ottawa

Hurwitz S 1981 Clinical pediatric dermatology. A textbook of skin disorders of childhood and adolescents. W B Saunders, Philadelphia

Jellard J 1957 Umbilical cord as a reservoir of infection in a maternity hospital. British Medical Journal   20: 925–28

Larson E 1987 Trends in neonatal infections. Journal of Obstetric, Gynecologic, and Neonatal Nursing   16: 404–09

Lawrence C 1982 Effect of two different methods of umbilical cord care on its separation time. Midwives Chronicle   95 (1134): 204–05

Martin G, Streng J, Miller M 1983 Current bathing techniques in newborn nurseries in the United States. American Journal of Diseases of Children 137: 529–30

Meberg A, Schøyen R 1985 Bacteriological colonization and neonatal infections. Acta Paediatrica Scandinavica   74: 366–71

Mugford M, Somchiwong M, Waterhouse I L 1986 Treatment of umbilical cords: a randomised trial to assess the effect of treatment methods on the work of midwives. Midwifery 2: 177–86

Murray M, Zentner J 1975 Nursing concepts for health promotion. Prentice Hall, New Jersey

Pildes R S, Ramamurthy R S, Vidyasagar D 1973 Effect of triple dye on staphylococcal colonization in the newborn infant. Pediatrics   82 (6): 987–90

Rush J 1986 Routine newborn bathing as a means of reducing *staphylococcus aureus* colonization rates: a randomized trial. Birth   13: 18–22

Rush J, Chalmers I, Enkin M 1989 Care of the new mother and baby. In Chalmers I, Enkin M, Kierse M (eds) Effective care in pregnancy and childbirth. Oxford University Press, Oxford

Salariya E M, Kowbus N M 1988 Variable cord care. Midwifery   4: 70–6

Schuman A J, Oksol B A 1985 The effect of isopropyl alcohol and triple dye on umbilical cord separation time. Military Medicine   150 (1): 49–50

Smith D H 1979 Epidemics of infectious diseases in newborn nurseries. Clinics in Obstetrics and Gynaecology   22 (2): 409–23

Speck W T, Driscoll J M, Polin R A, O'Neill J, Rosenkranz H S 1977 Staphylococcal and streptococcal colonization of the newborn infant. American Journal of Diseases of Children   131: 1005–08

Speck W T, Driscoll J M, O'Neill J, Rosenkranz H S 1980 Effect of antiseptic cord care on bacterial colonization in the newborn infant. Chemotherapy 26: 372–76

Stroud C E 1982 A pediatrician's view of the newborn and its epidemics. Current Medical Research and Opinion   7 (Supplement 2): 29–32

Wang E L, Elder D, Mishkel N 1987 Staphylococcal colonization and infection after discharge from a term newborn nursery. Infection Control   8 (Supplement 1): 30–3

Wilson C B, Ochs H D, Almquist J, Dassel S, Nauseth R, Ochs U H 1985 When is umbilical cord separation delayed? Journal of Pediatrics   107 (2): 292–94

Youmans G P, Patterson P Y, Sommers H M 1975 The bacteriological and clinical bases of infectious disease. W B Saunders, Philadelphia, Toronto

■ Further reading

Goldman D A 1981 Bacterial colonization and infection in the neonate. In Dixon R E (ed) Nosocomial infections. York Medical Books, Atlanta

Knapp R G 1978 Basic statistics for nurses. John Wiley, New York

Rush J, Chalmers I, Enkin M 1989 Care of the new mother and baby. In Chalmers I, Enkin M, Kierse M (eds) Effective care in pregnancy and childbirth. Oxford University Press, Oxford

Sackett D L, Haynes R B, Tugwell P 1985 Clinical epidemiology: a basic science for clinical medicine. Little, Brown & Co, Boston, Toronto

Young D 1982 Changing childbirth. Childbirth Graphics, Rochester NY

Chapter 6

Transitional care

Chris Whitby

In 1975 and 1978 respectively the maternity units in Exeter and Cambridge began to nurse low birthweight babies at their mothers' bedside. The babies normally weigh between 1.700 kg and 2.500 kg and are well at birth. This has become known as 'transitional care' or shared care with mothers.

It had long been the practice of neonatal units to admit routinely all babies weighing less than 2.500 kg at birth regardless of their condition. In the last 10 years the necessity for these admissions has been challenged, not only for small, well babies but for others such as babies born by forceps delivery, caesarean section, those needing phototherapy, small-for-dates babies and the babies of diabetic mothers (Brimblecombe *et al* 1978).

It is well recognised that babies and their parents benefit from early contact after birth (Kennell & Klaus 1982); with our increased knowledge and technology, it is now possible to differentiate between infants who require intensive or high dependency care and those who can benefit from transitional care.

The following are suggested advantages of transitional care:

1. Maternal/child attachment is facilitated if mother and baby are not separated. A possible reduction in non-accidental injury may result (Brimblecombe *et al* 1978);

2. Breastfeeding is more likely to succeed (de Cates *et al* 1982);

3. Babies can be discharged home earlier. Parents' confidence is increased, reducing management problems at home and the possible need for re-admission;

4. Communication between the midwifery department and the neonatal unit is improved;

5. Intensive care has developed very quickly over the last 10 years. The increasing survival rate of very small babies demands extra neonatal nursing time. Transitional care releases nursing resources for this purpose.

98

■ **It is assumed that you are already aware of the following:**

- The characteristics of the pre-term baby;
- The characteristics of the small-for-dates baby;
- The mechanisms of temperature control in the newborn;
- The principles of feeding low birthweight infants;
- The causes and management of neonatal hypoglycaemia.

■ **Transitional care**

During 1984–85 Jean Boxall (Exeter) and Chris Whitby (Cambridge) undertook a survey of transitional care (Boxall *et al* 1989). The senior nurses in charge of 351 British neonatal units were sent questionnaires; 251 of these were returned (a response rate of 71 per cent).

The questionnaires were used to collect a variety of relevant information, including size of unit and details of neonatal facilities. Nineteen maternity units (7.6 per cent) practising transitional care were identified. A further 17 units (6.8 per cent) were identified as caring for babies down to a birthweight of 1.8 kg in the normal postnatal wards. All of these hospitals were asked to complete a further questionnaire about the care mothers were allowed to give their babies and the facilities made available to them.

■ **Results**

□ **Criteria for admission to the neonatal unit**

Many infants are separated from their mothers and admitted to the neonatal unit because of local policy. Decisions regarding such admission are likely to be based on the babies' birthweight and gestation. Taking this into account, one of the questions in the survey asked specifically about the lowest weight at which infants might be admitted to the normal postnatal ward. Responses to this question indicated that 37 per cent of the hospitals surveyed will admit only infants weighing 2.2 kg or more to the normal ward.

A further question was concerned with the stage of gestation at which babies would be admitted to the postnatal ward with their mothers. Responses indicated that in 17 per cent of the hospitals surveyed, all infants of less than 37 weeks gestation were admitted to the neonatal unit.

Weight and gestation, however, are not the only criteria by which it is decided to separate babies from their mothers and nurse them in neonatal units. Other indications include a variety of medical conditions (affecting either the mother or the baby), and the necessity for treatments or procedures which are not available in the normal postnatal ward. Before 1987, it was also routine practice to admit all breech babies, and all those who had been delivered by caesarean section or forceps, to the neonatal unit for observation. The work of Brimblecombe *et al* (1978) suggested that any difficulties subsequently experienced by these babies and their parents were more likely to be due to the early separation than to the type of delivery. Policy has now changed in many hospitals and Boxall and colleagues' (1989) survey (see Table 6.1) found that only 4.5 per cent of units still use

Table 6.1 Numbers and percentage of hospitals with and without a transitional care facility where elective admission of babies to a neonatal unit has been thought to be necessary

| Separated care on a neonatal unit of ... | HOSPITALS | | | |
| | With transitional care | | Without transitional care | |
	No	%	*No*	%
Babies born by forceps	0/19	0	8/176*	4.5
Babies born by emergency LSCS	2/19	10	27/181	15
Babies born with Down's syndrome	0/19	0	9/177	5
Babies born with meconium stained liquor	3/19	16	37/178	20.7
Babies born to diabetic mothers	4/19	21	132/181	73

* The numbers in this column vary because not all hospitals taking part in the survey answered every question

forceps delivery as a criterion for separated special care. Those babies who are born with meconium stained liquor, or by caesarean section, are now more likely to be cared for on the postnatal ward with their mothers. The same would appear to apply to infants with Down's syndrome. The survey also indicated that 96.5 per cent of infants whose blood sugar levels need monitoring and 83 per cent of those requiring phototherapy are now nursed on the normal postnatal ward. The babies of diabetic mothers, however, are more likely to be cared for in the neonatal unit if transitional care is not available, as are infants requiring tube feeding and other procedures (see Table 6.2).

Table 6.2 Numbers and percentage of hospitals admitting babies to a neonatal unit for a required nursing procedure

| Separated care on a neonatal unit of babies requiring ... | HOSPITALS | | | |
| | With transitional care | | Without transitional care | |
	No	%	*No*	%
Phototherapy	0/19	0	32/186*	17
Blood sugar estimation	0/19	0	7/185	4
Incubator care	4/19	21	160/184	87
Tube feeding	0/19	0	129/185	70

* The numbers in this column vary because not all hospitals taking part in the survey answered every question

☐ **Facilities available and care given by mothers**

Answers to the survey questionnaires revealed that 19 of the hospitals contacted had specially designated areas providing transitional care. In addition, several senior nurses from neonatal units in other hospitals said that babies requiring transitional care were cared for on the normal post-natal ward by the same midwives who cared for the other mothers and babies (Cooke 1987). These two approaches to transitional care were compared and some interesting differences were revealed. As Table 6.3 makes clear, mothers in the normal wards are treated more as 'patients' than as parents. They have less freedom than their counterparts in the

Table 6.3 Visiting regulations and mothers' freedom to go out

	In transitional care N = 19		In normal wards N = 17	
Unrestricted visiting				
Fathers	16	84.21	11	64.7
Siblings	16	84.21	9	52.94
Grandparents	13	68.42	8	47.06
Others	9	47	6	35.29
Mothers can go shopping	18	94.74	10	58.32
Mothers can go out for a meal	15	78.95	9	52.4

Table 6.4 Care given by parents

	In transitional care N = 19		In normal ward N = 17	
	No	%	No	%
Tube feeding	18	94.74	9	52.94
Incubator care	17	89.47	7	41.18
Respiratory monitoring	17	89.47	6	35.29

transitional care areas. As the table also shows, the attitude to other family members appears to be more relaxed in the transitional care areas than in the postnatal wards.

■ Transitional care: some guidelines

Transitional care is being organised in three ways. In the first instance, a separate postnatal ward, staffed by midwives, supervised by paediatricians and the senior neonatal nurse/midwife, is set aside for this type of care. Alternatively, care is given by the neonatal unit staff in the unit's mother and baby rooms and/or on an adjacent postnatal ward. The third possibility is that babies down to a birthweight of 1.800 kg are cared for in the normal postnatal wards.

Midwives are well able to care for these mothers and babies and organisation of care by neonatal unit staff is rare. The babies are not sick, and it is not necessary to employ neonatal nurses whose expertise is best used in caring for the sick babies. Midwives will, however, need in-service training, support and advice, probably from the neonatal unit senior nurse and/or sisters. Guidelines for care should be drawn up as described below.

Midwifery staffing levels need not differ from other postnatal wards if these mothers are totally involved in the care of their babies. Support workers are necessary however, and there may be a role for the nursery nurse in transitional care wards.

Whichever way a particular hospital decides to organise care, there are several important clinical considerations.

□ Criteria for admission

These should be clearly defined and paediatricians should ensure that only fit, warm babies are admitted for transitional care. The babies are usually of a gestational age greater than 32 weeks and of a birthweight between 1.700 kg and 2.500 kg.

Babies of this birthweight and above, who needed to be admitted to the neonatal unit at birth but have recovered from their illness, can be transferred to the ward to be looked after by their mothers.

Babies with malformations which are not life-threatening, such as cleft lip and palate, Down's syndrome or spina bifida, can also be nursed in a transitional care ward.

☐ Temperature control

All newborn babies chill quickly after birth if allowed to do so. We rely heavily on good practices in the delivery unit to ensure that pre-term babies do not lose body heat excessively at birth and are delivered to the transitional care ward in good condition. The following measures can be taken:

- Make sure the delivery room is warm, close the windows and add heating if necessary;

- Use a resuscitaire with overhead heater and make sure this is turned on a good half-hour before the baby's birth;

- Receive the baby into warm wraps, dry him thoroughly, remove the wet wraps and replace them with warm dry ones;

- Keep the baby covered as much as possible while resuscitation is being undertaken;

- When the parents have seen and held their baby and he has been dressed using a hat, bootees and cardigan, transfer him to the transitional care ward as soon as possible.

The baby should be nursed in the ward nursery until his temperature is normal (37°C). The use of clothing – stretch suits, bonnets, bootees and woollen jackets – is recommended. Cot lids are also useful. When the ambient temperature cannot be raised sufficiently, a free standing heater next to the cot works very well. Incubators may be used occasionally but are usually unnecessary.

☐ Phototherapy

Phototherapy can be given in the postnatal ward nursery where heating is adequate. Incubators can be used. Most mothers, given the choice of phototherapy in an incubator at their bedside or in a cot in the neonatal unit, choose the former.

☐ **Feeding and blood sugar**

All pre-term and small babies should have their blood sugar measured using BM or Dextrostix within two hours after birth. The babies, including those to be breastfed subsequently, should be fed early (that is, at two hours) using a formula milk (pre-term babies must continue to receive adequate calories for growth and steady weight gain throughout this period). If the first blood sugar measurement is low (less than 1 mmol/litre) the baby should be fed with a pre-term formula and the paediatrician informed (Pildes *et al* 1974; de Cates *et al* 1982). If the baby is asymptomatic, it is likely that the blood sugar will be checked after one hour. If it remains less than 1 mmol/litre it is probable that intravenous therapy will be necessary even if the baby is asymptomatic. (Symptoms suggestive of hypoglycaemia are pallor, floppiness, vomiting, a tendency towards jitteriness, and apnoea.) If the first blood sugar is between 1–2 mmol/litre the baby should be fed by nasogastric tube and the level checked after three hours. If it remains between 1–2 mmol/litre a true measurement of the blood sugar level may be taken, the baby fed again and the results of the test awaited. Then the paediatrician will decide whether further treatment is necessary.

Lucas *et al* (1988) suggested that low blood sugar measurements for more than three days may cause adverse neurodevelopmental outcome. If kept warm and well fed, however, most of these small, well babies achieve good blood sugar levels (2–3 mmol/litre) within 24 hours of birth.

Babies should be fed sufficient amounts of milk per kilo of body weight. More detailed guidelines are given in Table 6.5. Usually blood sugar estimation will be undertaken six hourly for 48 hours and babies fed regularly three hourly.

In looking at the Cambridge transitional care ward (de Cates *et al* 1982) a very low incidence of asymptomatic hypoglycaemia was reported and a complete absence of symptomatic hypoglycaemia in a large number (167) of small-for-dates infants who were fed early and screened for low blood sugar. Small-for-dates babies may want bigger feeds, starting at 90 mls/kg/day, always remaining one day ahead on the feeding regimen described in Table 6.5. Small babies will not usually be able to sustain sucking in order to complete feeds and should not be tired out by being forced to do so.

Table 6.5 Recommended amounts of milk for babies to be fed per kilo of body weight

Day 1	60 ml/kg/day
Day 2	90 ml/kg/day
Day 3	120 ml/kg/day
Day 4	150 ml/kg/day
Day 7	180 ml/kg/day
Day 10	200 ml/kg/day

Supplementary feeding by nasogastric tube should be undertaken until the baby is able to suck sufficiently on the breast or bottle. Mothers should be taught to tube feed so that they can take total care of the baby under the supervision of the nurse or midwife.

Breastfeeding can be encouraged and the baby put to the breast as often as possible without tiring him. Full tube feeds should continue until the baby is obviously taking milk from the breast, then the tube feeds can be reduced by 5 or 10 mls. If the baby continues to gain weight daily this weaning process continues until the baby is fully breastfed, but this may take some time to achieve.

After initial loss, weight gain should be steady and recorded daily. Any loss of more than 100 g in 24 hours should be reported to the paediatrician.

□ Infection control

The usual local infection control policies should be adhered to. All parents and visitors should be properly instructed in hand washing. The neonatal unit hand washing policies should be extended to the transitional care ward or area.

The two most important factors in the prevention of infection are good hand washing practices (Lowbury *et al* 1974) and allowing the mother to care for her own baby (Haley & Bregman 1982). This reduces the number of people handling him, and so minimises the chances of cross infection.

Good techniques and thorough cleansing of equipment should continue. Nurses, doctors or visitors with infections should not handle infants, in particular if they have colds, coughs, diarrhoea or vomiting, infected lesions (such as oral herpes) or fevers. Infected mothers and babies should be nursed in a single room. Baby clothes and woollens should be washed in a machine, not by hand, in order to ensure adequate water temperatures.

Providing the points above are considered, an increase in infection should not be expected. A retrospective study undertaken in Exeter since the evolvement of transitional care (Boxall *et al* 1982) has shown a drop in local infections (of the eye, skin and umbilical cord for example) despite there having been no change in cleansing techniques or antibiotic policy.

□ Length of stay

The average length of stay in the Cambridge unit is 10 days. However the smaller babies may be in for 21 days. Most mothers who are involved in the care of the baby will stay, but after seven days it is good for morale to encourage them to get up and dressed, and to go out for short periods between feeds. Some mothers will have been in hospital for long periods antenatally and need these short breaks, especially if the baby's stay does stretch to three weeks.

■ Recommendations for clinical practice

1. Transitional care or shared care with mothers should be made available across the UK to all mothers with well pre-term or low dependency special care babies.

2. The goal should be to involve mothers in their own infant's care as soon after birth as possible. When encouraged to do this, mothers are able to take over total infant care earlier and as a result will build up their confidence and be able to take their babies home sooner.

3. Midwives are encouraged to participate in this care in collaboration with the neonatal nurses and paediatricians.

4. This initiative should not be used simply as a means of releasing staff for intensive care or delivery suites.

■ Practice check

- What measures are taken in your maternity unit to keep mothers and their babies together whenever possible?

- What is the admission policy for the neonatal unit/SCBU in your hospital?

- Is there a paediatrician available for every pre-term or difficult birth?

- Is there a transitional care ward or area?

- Do you think that the care of small, well babies and their mothers should be a part of normal postnatal care, or organised as a separate ward/area and staffed from the neonatal unit?

- If your neonatal unit/SCBU *routinely* admits babies who are not sick or very small (even for a few hours), can you challenge this policy?

□ Acknowledgements

Tables 6.1–6.4 inclusive, as well as the 'Recommendations for clinical practice' on page 106, are all taken or adapted from the article by Boxall J, Lawrence C, Tripp J, Whitby C (1989) 'Who is holding the baby?' which appeared in the *Midwives Chronicle* 102 (1213). Thanks are due to the *Midwives Chronicle* for permission to use this material.
    The study on which the above article and part of this chapter are based was funded by the Iolanthe Trust – which also provided the funding for a

teaching video on transitional care. The video is entitled 'Being together' and is available to hire from the Neonatal Nurses' Association, A Block, Forest House, Berkeley Avenue, Nottingham MG3 5AF, or to buy from Line-Up, Freshford, Bath BA3 6BX.

■ References

Boxall J, Cruickshank J G, Orme R L E 1982 Shared care and infection in special care baby units. Nursing Times 78 (44): 1848–50

Boxall J, Lawrence C, Tripp J, Whitby C 1989 Who is holding the baby? Midwives Chronicle 102 (1213): 34–6

Brimblecombe F S W, Richards M P M, Roberton N R C 1978 Separation and special care baby units: 12–29. Spastics International Medical Publications. Heinemann, London

Cooke R W I, Weindling A M 1987 Establishment of an intermediate care ward for mothers and babies. Archives of Disease in Childhood 62: 1198

de Cates C R, Whitby C, Roberton N R C 1982 Infants weighing 1.8 kg to 2.5 kg – should they be cared for in neonatal units or on post-natal wards? Lancet i: 322

Haley R W, Bregman D A 1982 The role of understaffing and overcrowding in recurrent outbreaks of staphylococcal infection in a neonatal special care nursery. Journal of Infectious Diseases 145: 875–85

Kennell J H, Klaus M H 1982 Parent-infant bonding. Mosby, St Louis

Lowbury B J L, Lilly H A, Ayliffe G A J 1974 The use of alcohol solutions of disinfectants on the skin flora. British Medical Journal iv: 369

Lucas A, Morley R, Cole J J 1988 Adverse neurodevelopmental outcome of moderate neonatal hypoglycaemia. British Medical Journal 297: 1304–08

Pildes R S, Cornblath M, Warren I, Page-El I, Di Menza S, Merritt D M, Peeva A 1974 A prospective controlled study of neonatal hypoglycaemia. Pediatrics 54: 5

■ Suggested further reading

Boxall J, Lawrence C, Tripp J, Whitby C 1989 Who is holding the baby? Midwives Chronicle 102 34–6

Brimblecombe F S W, Richards M P M, Roberton N R C 1978 Separation and special care baby units. Spastics International Medical Publications. Heinemann, London

Davis J A, Richards M P M, Roberton N R C (eds) 1983 Parent-baby attachment in premature infants. Croom Helm, London

Green A, Sultiész G 1985 Hypoglycaemia in infancy and childhood. Churchill Livingstone, Edinburgh

Harvey D 1987 Parent-infant relationships. John Wiley, Chichester

Chapter 7

Care of the grieving parent with special reference to stillbirth

Margaret Adams and Joyce Prince

The perinatal mortality rate for England and Wales in 1988 was 8.7 for every 1000 live and stillbirths (OPCS 1988). The risk of perinatal death is higher for multiple births (McMullan 1986) and for babies in neonatal units (HC 1980). Parents who have decided on a therapeutic abortion have a painful path to tread and they too will need support in their loss, as will parents who suffer a spontaneous abortion. A midwife should be prepared therefore to help those parents who have lost their baby, either through neonatal death, stillbirth or abortion. The handicapped baby may also precipitate a sense of loss because the imagined 'perfect child' (Gardner 1986) will not materialise. In some instances, the mother may go home while her handicapped, sick or premature baby remains behind in the neonatal unit. The longed for perfect child is mourned while parents try to care for and love the defective baby for which they were not prepared. Their contact with the child does help to make him a 'real person'. Mourning is generally found to be easier when there is a recognised focus for grief (Newman 1984), so that when death does occur the grieving process may be managed to give more effective resolution.

A sense of loss may be experienced too by parents who have set their hearts on having a child of one sex and who find themselves with the opposite one. Neither should it be forgotten that the decision by a single mother to have her baby adopted is likely to be extremely painful.

Parental grief is an important topic and one which deserves to be explored fully. As there is not sufficient space here to cover all aspects, this chapter will concentrate mainly on stillbirth. Midwives should be familiar, however, with grief in other situations (see 'Suggested further reading' page 123). They should give serious thought to how they will handle the grief response if it arises unexpectedly – during the antenatal booking interview for example.

108

■ It is assumed that you are already aware of the following:

- That there is a large body of work on grief and bereavement, beginning with the work of Kubler-Ross (1970) and Murray Parkes (1972);

- The basic skills needed for counselling, and how to make effective use of them;

- The specialist counselling services available in your area (including local branches of organisations such as SANDS, the Miscarriage Association and Relate, as well as any services provided by your health authority) and how to refer clients to them should it be necessary.

■ Death and grief

Today, the great majority of deaths take place in hospital and are regarded by health professionals and the public alike as manifestations of failure (Kubler-Ross 1970). Considerable energy and resources are spent on physical efforts to avoid death 'prematurely' while psychological and emotional aspects of the failure to do so seem to be little understood. Death is often lonely and impersonal, both for the dying person and for the bereaved relative and friends. The hospice movement has helped to make good an important gap in the health service for the adult terminally ill, but the trauma to parents and family occasioned by death at, or before, birth has yet to attract a comparable development.

The normal stages of grief as described by Kubler-Ross (1970) are as follows. Initially there is a numbness, in which the death is acknowledged intellectually but there is an absence of appropriate feeling. The person may feel as if he or she is 'in a dream'. This is followed by disbelief and then the onset of acute grief in which the pain of loss is experienced. The need to signal the pain may emerge in the form of crying or shouting, and there may also be a searching for the dead person. Anger is often a prominent feature – anger with the deceased for leaving, anger with professionals for failure or neglect, anger with God for letting it happen, anger with themselves in the form of guilt. Maturation of the bereaved personality and adjustment to the loss leads eventually to acceptance. Other authorities (Parkes 1972; Tschudin 1987) concur on the sequence of the stages. Their duration varies and there may be delay in working through any of them. Suppression at any stage may cause chronic or pathological grief and the risk of psychiatric difficulties (Engel 1962).

The majority of deaths occur after a life lasting many years but, although both stillbirths and neonatal deaths have been reduced dramatically during this century, a baby may die before it is viable, before labour, during labour or after it has lived and breathed independently of its mother. There is a particular poignancy about death which occurs before, or very soon after, extrauterine life has begun. It brings particular problems to the mourning and grieving process, as there is very little to remember about the life that has gone (Kennell *et al* 1970). The parents are unprepared for sadness as they and their friends were anticipating the celebration of a joyful event. When the 'grief work' or mourning process is interrupted (as may happen if a new pregnancy occurs), or if grief is pathological, difficulties may be projected onto other children in the family. Bourne and Lewis (1984) found that parents whose grief was unresolved were more likely to have difficulty in managing the next baby and that there was an increased risk of its being abused or rejected.

It should not be forgotten that staff have needs too. The midwife who has supported grieving parents, counselled those whose antenatal investigations have revealed a handicapped fetus, or who has delivered a baby that has subsequently died, may need to come to terms with her own sense of disappointment and sorrow. There is much to be said for the maintenance of a staff support and discussion group (Roch 1987) which should perhaps be run by a behavioural scientist or therapist with experience in group work.

☐ **Death before life begins: miscarriage and therapeutic abortion**

Many women whose pregnancies end well before the 28th week of gestation will not receive midwifery care at all around that time. As a result, some midwives may feel that it is unnecessary to concern themselves with this issue. In an article entitled 'Forgotten women' (Moore 1987), one midwife lays down an impassioned challenge to this viewpoint:

> The World Health Organisation states that the midwife is qualified to care for women at any stage of pregnancy. Is it fair, then, to reject these women as the failures they so often feel themselves to be?

Even if all midwives do not subscribe to Moore's view, they should be aware that the questions asked about previous pregnancies at the antenatal booking interview may well reopen old wounds (Methven 1982). They should also be aware that women whose grief or guilt for an earlier pregnancy is still unresolved may be at greater than average risk of developing postnatal depression (Kumar & Robson 1978; Paykel *et al* 1980; Gibbons 1984; see also Chapter 3 in this volume, 'Emotional problems associated with childbirth).

Approximately 80 per cent of spontaneous abortions occur in the first trimester. Society accords the event no recognition through ritual or expression of sympathy (Alexander 1984). Yet for both parents and professionals, a sense of failure is often keenly felt. It is generally conceded that the expression, rather than suppression, of feelings is part of the process of coming to terms with loss. Parents need to have the opportunity to review their emotions and attitudes with an empathic professional person.

Assumptions about whether or not an individual woman regards her fetus as an actual baby, before it is recognisable to anyone else as such, can be unwise. Certainly to Karen Nash (1987), a midwife and mother whose third pregnancy aborted at 11 weeks, 'Its still a baby', and although her account is entirely subjective, this attitude is supported by research. For example, Pepper and Knapp (1980) found that the reactions of women who suffer fetal loss are similar to those who suffer stillbirth or neonatal death. The survey by Oakley *et al* (1990), although open to criticism for its use of a self-selected sample, indicates that the level of grief and loss experienced by women after miscarriage is not only very high, but is also largely ignored by health professionals.

Therapeutic abortion for fetal abnormality is usually carried out well into the second trimester. By this time, the woman is likely to be visibly pregnant and may have felt the baby move. Second trimester terminations are usually preceded by some careful assessments and, probably, a difficult and painful decision on the part of the parents. The role of the midwife can be a crucial one in this situation (Kenyon 1988). Follow-up counselling may also be necessary as, no matter how 'sensible' her decision appears, the woman may later suffer greatly. Penson (1990) describes a personal encounter with a 41 year old woman whose grief and guilt caught up with her once the decision and the termination were behind her. She is quoted as saying:

> It was my baby, and I killed it. I committed murder. They say he would have been very handicapped, but how can they know how bad he would have been ... I loved him, he was mine, and I allowed them to take him away from me.

Any pregnancy with an outcome other than a live, healthy baby is likely to lead to parental guilt and anxiety that may be reactivated during a subsequent pregnancy (Methven 1982). The midwife who is able to encourage some discussion of these feelings is likely to provide considerable help towards their resolution (Tom-Johnson 1990). An area that may be particularly difficult to address is that of therapeutic abortion for reasons that are primarily social or psychological. Neustatter and Newson (1986) found that this is a subject associated with particular shame and distress on the part of many women, who may have kept the incident secret for many years. Webb's work (1985a, 1985b) shed a disturbing light on the attitudes of nurses towards women undergoing or known to have undergone termination of pregnancy, suggesting that they were hostile, judgemental or created 'barriers to sympathy'. Midwives should be aware of these findings and consider carefully what the implications might be for their own practice.

■ Stillbirth: a critical appraisal of the literature

The literature on loss, death, grief and bereavement is extensive. There is much that is movingly written from first hand experience (for example, Hill 1989). Descriptive material in the professional press is very valuable in heightening awareness of the difficulties faced by the bereaved parent. Systematic enquiry can be found in the large sociological survey report in the Perinatal Mortality Survey (Butler & Bonham 1963) and in Perinatal Problems (Butler 1969) (this uses data from a much larger national survey of all births in one week in 1958). These surveys indicate that perinatal death is more common in the lower socioeconomic groups, at the extremes of the child bearing age, or among illegitimate births. The likelihood is, therefore, that a perinatal death will occur in already disadvantaged families. Small scale studies (some of which are described below) have taken the form of assessing the reactions of bereft parents, of evaluating their management and assessing their short and long term needs. These studies have, of necessity, used only small numbers of people. When a sample is restricted there is much to be said for precise replication so that a more reliable information base can be built up. This has not been done. Parental bereavement is intrinsically a difficult matter to research. In addition to the small numbers involved, the topic is a highly emotional one and the parents themselves are initially in a state of shock. The situation is novel and therefore the language with which to communicate is not readily available either to parents or to staff. Follow up may be confounded by the wish of parents not to reactivate painful memories.

Comments on the deficiencies of the small scale research reports that are available must be seen in the light of these inherent difficulties. The failure of some professional journals to have a proper refereeing system for research papers does nothing to improve the reliability of the knowledge base on which, increasingly, professionals are trying to base their work.

One of the earliest relevant studies was by Giles (1970) who investigated 40 bereaved women and found their physical and emotional reactions similar to the classical descriptions of grief for loss of an adult, as had been made by Lindman (1944) and Kubler-Ross (1970). Culberg (1972) studied 56 mothers and showed, like Giles, that pathological grief may develop where the normal grieving process has been delayed. Bereavement counselling was claimed to be effective by Parkes (1980) and others, but there have been inadequate controlled trials. Forrest *et al* (1982) tested the hypothesis that psychological recovery from stillbirth or neonatal death is enhanced by a planned programme of support and counselling. Twenty five mothers of stillbirths and twenty five of neonatal deaths entered the controlled trial where they were randomly allocated to receive either planned support or routine care. The two groups were comparable in respect of age, social class, previous obstetric history, and method of delivery. Thirteen of the stillbirths were macerated and seven had congenital abnormalities. The effect of this on the parents as compared to those with neonatal deaths was not explored. Both parents in the planned programme were counselled by either a social worker, if the family was known to one, or by a midwife. Details of the counsellors are not given, nor is it reported whether the midwives were trained as counsellors. Evaluation was, however, undertaken blindly by a trained interviewer conducting a semi-structured interview six and fourteen months after the death. Two self rating scales measuring psychiatric disturbance were also used.

At six months, 30 per cent of the sample had dropped out of the study, and by 14 months this had increased to 40 per cent. Fewer mothers in the supported group showed psychiatric disorder at the six month interview, but by 14 months there was no significant difference. The conclusion drawn is that recovery is facilitated by support and counselling. The lack of a supportive network of friends and neighbours and lack of a warm intimate free relationship with her partner were identified as considerable 'risk factors' for the mother. Raw figures of some factors used in the analysis are not given. It seems likely that the total sample size is insufficient to support any general conclusion on these matters, and replication of the work would be useful.

Certain ways to facilitate grieving were suggested:

- Supportive care and counselling;

- Discussion with medical staff about what went wrong;

- Support for parents after discharge by relevant voluntary and statutory community services;

- A delay of six months before starting another pregnancy.

A similar study was conducted by White *et al* (1984) with 12 families whose babies had died in the special care nursery at Stobhill Hospital, Glasgow. The purpose was to see if the handling according to specified recommendations was being achieved, and if it was what the parents wanted. Interviews with the 12 families took place from 2–13 months after the death, and, as might be expected, they presented a heterogeneous picture. It was evident that the needs of the parents were highly individual, and that there was room for improvement in the management of the problem. As a result of the study a check list for completion after the death of a baby was designed so that oversights and replications might be reduced or avoided.

A variety of articles suggesting interventions for aiding the bereaved have been published in the USA. These articles are based on opinion, however, rather than research. Lake *et al* (1983) point out that there is a 'singular need to document the clinical effectiveness of such' programmes.

An attempt to evaluate midwifery care for the mother of the stillborn baby was carried out at Queen Charlotte's Hospital by Gohlish (1985). This was a small exploratory study. Thirty statements descriptive of helpful behaviour were derived from research literature, and the research objective was to put these behaviours into rank order from most to least helpful in terms of support, comfort and facilitating grieving. The plan was to interview all nineteen mothers who delivered a stillbirth during 1982/3. Fifteen were contacted, five could not participate, and of the remaining ten, four were so obviously in need of immediate counselling that they had to be excluded from the sample. The six remaining identified seven statements as helpful. These were:

- The midwife should recognise when the mother wished to talk about her baby;

- The mother should be allowed to decide the length of time she stayed in hospital;

- The mother should be allowed to choose whether she was in a single room or in the main ward;

- The mother should be asked whether she would like a photograph of the baby;

- The mother should be informed that she could see the baby, even after several days;

- Analgesia should be given as needed;

- The mother should be informed that lactation would occur.

The specific purpose of the research was not achieved but enough information emerged to lead to a change in postmortem and burial procedures, and the development of a checklist for use after delivery. These changes have yet to be evaluated.

The centenary of the Royal College of Midwives was celebrated by having special issues of the Midwives Chronicle. One issue (August 1987), carried several articles on bereavement, including the report of an enquiry into the best management for the mother of a stillbirth by Hughes (1987). Thirteen mothers were interviewed (by whom and how is not revealed). The time since the stillbirth was three days to 20 years. Inaccuracy of recall over long periods renders some of the data questionable. In addition, there have been considerable changes of policy and practice over 20 years which makes for further methodological muddle. A plea for improvement in communication is the suitably bland outcome of this diffuse study. Rice (1982) and Gohlish (1985) have also identified the need for good and accurate communication in caring for the bereaved parents. There is a general need amongst midwives to develop their social and interactive skills as shown by Adams (1987) who studied the communication in the normal second stage of labour.

■ Intrauterine death: some practical suggestions

Despite the paucity of research on this matter there are some suggestions for practice that seem sensible and kind.

An honest explanation of the cause of death (if it is known), the likely course of labour and delivery should be made by the obstetrician and/or the paediatrician to both parents. Some discussion about the way the baby is to be treated and the parent's wishes in this regard should follow. This should be done in the presence of an experienced midwife so that she can, if necessary, continue any discussion to clarify points that may not have been understood or accepted. Bereavement can put a very great strain on a relationship. There may be anger, resentment, guilt, disappointment and the apportionment of blame. The midwife can perform a very important function if she can help the parents to discuss together frankly without thinking they have to protect each other or disguise their feelings from one another (Alexander 1984; Kohner 1985; Hutti 1988). The considerable task of re-organising themselves psychologically will lie ahead, for which deception will not form a good foundation. All staff on duty in the area must be made aware of the death and the parents should not be left alone unless they wish to be.

□ Labour

Generous pain relief should be offered, and given to the mother (if she wishes it). *Full* midwifery care is needed. The use of medical or esoteric terminology should be avoided and clear explanations should be given and repeated (Forrest *et al* 1982). An assessment of the parents' understanding of events should be made from time to time.

Inexperienced staff should not be left unsupported, and anyone who has herself suffered a recent bereavement may be particularly vulnerable. The delivery itself needs sensitive handling and this is more likely to be achieved by a midwife with some previous relevant experience. Bereavement workshops with an experiential component in counselling can give vital insight to those who have little experience and additional help to those who have more, as individuals vary so much in their reactions. A stillbirth produces an unmanageable conflict of feelings and confusion about the whole process of birth and death. Instrumental delivery, especially under general anaesthetic can cause further bewilderment and anxiety (Bourne & Lewis 1984). Women have felt the needlessness of the wounds and the stigma of becoming a surgical patient instead of a mother. If the baby can be delivered normally that is certainly the course to be recommended.

Some mothers delivered of a macerated stillbirth, have apparently been surprised by the fact that the baby's body is still whole. It would be wise to ensure that the mother is aware of this before the labour begins.

The baby who dies during labour presents the shock of sudden death. The parents have had no time to consider that death rather than new life awaits them. Staff will also be dismayed and there is absolutely no harm in them showing their own sorrow. Professionals sometimes distract themselves with unnecessary business. All the indications are that mothers would prefer someone just to sit quietly with them, listening as necessary (Kohner 1985).

☐ Care of the dead baby

In view of the need in the grief process to acknowledge the dead person it is important that the parents should have some real experience of their baby. Past practice has often been to remove the dead child and not to allow the parents to see or hold it. It is likely that this is harmful in that it colludes in the disbelief stage and distorts or delays the grieving process.

Mothers would like their baby to be treated like any other – that is, wrapped up and given to them to hold if they wish, or dressed when they are ready. Photographs can be taken – where possible these should be slides or snaps rather than polaroid pictures, as the latter tend to fade. Skilled photography can help bring out the best and camouflage the less normal features where the baby is abnormal or macerated. The baby, though dead, has been a living being for several months and has been the focus for plans and hopes. His dying may seem all the more desperate if no recognition is given of his brief existence. Talking about the baby – his size, his sex and who he resembles – may help to make the event more real to the parents so that their grief can be focused. Momentos such as a lock of hair, a footprint, tape measure, cot card and identification band are tangible reminders of the baby's existence. They are all there is to show, with photographs, to relatives and friends.

☐ Care of the mother

The midwife can help the parents decide where the mother would prefer to be nursed if there is a choice. Gohlish (1985) found that the opportunity to decide this was much appreciated. Not all mothers want to be in a single room (Hughes 1987). If a bereaved mother so chooses (and the other mothers are willing), the midwife could go with her and introduce her to the ward staff and to other mothers who are sometimes pleased to talk. This may help to make the event more significant. Such situations, however, must be handled with tact. Some new mothers – particularly if they are superstitious – may prefer to avoid the bereaved parent and staff should be sensitive to the feelings of all involved.

Wherever the bereaved mother is nursed, her friends and family members may be able to give support if visiting times can be modified.

Mothers who have lost their babies are frequently surprised – and distressed – to find they start lactating. They should be warned about this and also included in all the postnatal exercises that are done in the ward. Inexperienced staff may think that sedation would be helpful but most women would rather face the pain of bereavement than delay it. Listening to the mother, especially when she talks about her labour, is greatly appreciated. She may go over the same ground many times in her search for meaning and order. Constant repetition of the same question – despite a comprehensive reply – may indicate a deeper unarticulated problem which needs sensitive exploration.

□ Special cases

When one twin dies or is stillborn, the parents have to celebrate life and death together. Mothers of twins find this is so hard that they may become alienated from the living child as they either resent its continued life or think it does not compare favourably with the idealised dead 'angel' baby (Lewis & Bryan 1988). The survivor can feel very lonely and also guilty for being alive if this issue has not been resolved by the parents within a few months. Such parents have special needs and can meet others in a similar position through the Twins and Multiple Births Association (TAMBA). For further reading on the special problems associated with multiple pregnancy, the reader is referred to the chapter by Jane Spillman in the volume in this series on 'Antenatal Care'.

□ Arrangements for burial

The midwife needs to ensure that the relevant regulations have been complied with and that parents are informed about procedures. Much trauma is caused if registry office officials express any doubt as to the veracity of the parents' statements. If the child has lived at all, both a birth and a death certificate are required and a medical practitioner must sign these. A doctor or a midwife may sign the stillbirth certificate and the UKCC (1989) Midwife's Code of Practice gives details about this.

It is the duty of the parent(s) to present the relevant certificates at the office of the Registrar of Births, Marriages and Deaths of the district in which the child is born. It is helpful to telephone the office before the father goes to register the death so that he can avoid waiting among the other parents. It may also be advisable to see that he is accompanied. A certificate of registration of stillbirth can be given to the parents by the registrar and this can perhaps provide the comfort of some kind of official acknowledgement that their baby existed.

The parents have to decide whether arrangements for the burial shall be made by the hospital or privately, and whether they wish to have a private grave or one which ultimately will contain more than one coffin. A private grave can be permanently marked. Some parents have found that the place of burial is important to them and they should be aware that a shared grave cannot be marked. It would be helpful for parents to be told what charges are made for these services by the hospital and the local undertaker.

The body of a stillborn baby cannot be moved from the hospital mortuary without a certificate of disposal which must be issued by the registrar of births and deaths on receipt of the certificate of stillbirth.

If cremation has been chosen, a certificate with signatures of two medical practitioners must be completed. The parents also need to decide whether or not they wish to have a religious service to mark the burial or cremation. The midwife working in a multi-cultural area will need to be able to help as necessary by contacting the appropriate religious leader and local funeral director who can make all the arrangements.

The obstetrician or paediatrician may wish to have parental permission for a post mortem examination. The midwife should be present at the discussion so that she can clarify any issues that have not been fully understood. It is generally the case that parents accede to this request as they particularly want to know why their baby died. The Third Report of the Maternity Services Advisory Committee (1985) says 'Parents should be given as much information as possible on the cause of their baby's death, be encouraged to discuss it and advised of any implication for the future'. The benefits of having a proper funeral for a stillbirth, which can be arranged by the hospital contractor for a small fee, may not be realised by the parents. It provides a focus for them, for the grandparents, friends and perhaps most important, other children that they may have. Goodall (1984) found that children who have not been involved in discussions about a dead sibling, and who are protected from the impact that the death makes, may develop bizarre ideas about him or her which can have disrupting effects on their behaviour possibly persisting for years.

☐ **Going home**

It used to be common practice to send the mother home as quickly as possible. This may not, however, be in her best interest. Discussion with her about her home support is vital. Those who are in any way isolated, or who have an unsupportive partner, can be referred for bereavement counselling, as these are the groups identified by Forrest *et al* (1982) and by White *et al* (1984) as being at risk in developing pathological grief reactions. Careful communication with the community midwife and health visitor can avoid the faux pas made in ignorance, which may add greatly to the parents' distress.

Family planning can be discussed when appropriate as authorities generally agree that six months to one year is necessary to complete the grieving process (Bourne & Lewis 1984). Literature can often be helpful as the parents can pick it up and read it when they feel ready. Many institutions have their own booklet on stillbirth and there are helpful notes and pamphlets available nationally.

Follow up either by a local counsellor or a bereavement team member (Gohlish 1985) could be helpful, though the effectiveness of these has nowhere been evaluated. Support groups such as the Stillbirth and Neonatal Death Association (SANDS) have often been found to be helpful. The telephone number of the local group can be given to the mother when she is discharged. The Irish branch of SANDS has produced a booklet *A Little Lifetime* which parents may find useful. Demeaning the significance of the lost baby (for example, 'you can always try again' or 'at least you have other children' is to be avoided).

Bourne and Lewis (1984) advised on care being taken not to overlook a previous loss when a further pregnancy is established. Continuity from the obstetric team – and particularly the midwife – is ideal so that the sensitivities associated with the previous loss are properly understood. In this way, the woman may be helped to enjoy her later, successful pregnancy rather than it providing occasion for her to relive previous sorrow.

■ Recommendations for clinical practice

1. Antenatal booking interviews should be undertaken by experienced midwives with a knowledge of counselling skills. Adequate time should be allowed at booking for women to talk freely and express their feelings about previous terminations or reproductive casualties.

2. Anniversaries of previous neonatal or cot deaths should be recorded in the woman's notes so that staff involved in her care are aware that they must be particularly sensitive to her emotional needs on these dates.

3. Continuity of care should be provided for women going into labour following an intrauterine death. This planning should take into account the value of periodic breaks for the midwife who is looking after the woman.

4. Parents should be given as much information as is known about the cause of their baby's death. They should be made to feel that the staff realise the significance of their loss. They should be consulted and their wishes respected over how the dead baby should be managed. Staff should take care to handle the baby as carefully as they would if he were alive.

5. Parents should be given the opportunity to hold and cuddle their dead baby. They should be given the opportunity to spend some time alone with him and arrangements should be made for photographs of the baby to be taken so that they may have some tangible momento.

6. Whenever possible, the mother should be consulted about whether she would prefer to be lodged in a side room or on the ward. If she wishes her partner to stay with her, arrangements should be made for this also. The feelings of other mothers on the ward should also be taken into account.

7. It should not be forgotten that fathers are also bereaved and that, even though they feel they should appear strong for their partner's sake, they may also need support and counselling.

8. If the baby is born alive but not expected to live long, parents should be given every opportunity to participate in his care and to get to know him.

■ Practice check

- When taking a woman's history, do you make use of the different types of question used in counselling skills?

- Do you encourage the woman who has had an intrauterine death to make active choices about her labour – what position to adopt, what level/type of analgesia she would prefer, whether she wishes her partner to be present etc?

- Do you feel able to show parents whose baby has been born handicapped, sick or dead that you are saddened too?

- Do you give the bereaved parents the time and space to talk about what has happened as they try to make sense of their tragedy?

- Do you attempt to answer parents' questions as sensitively and honestly as you can? Do you avoid technical language and jargon?

- What provisions are there in your unit for parents to be involved in the care of a severely handicapped or dying baby? What support is available for such parents?

- Are you familiar with the legal requirements that have to be fulfilled before burial or cremation can take place? Do you know what decisions the parents of a dead baby will have to make before the body can be cremated or buried?

- In the case of miscarriage, termination for fetal abnormality, stillbirth or neonatal death, what arrangements are there for liaison and exchange of information with community staff to ensure that the parents receive continuity of care after transfer home?

- Is the protocol of your hospital satisfactory? If not, what improvements can you suggest?

- Is there a support group available for staff? If not, should you be thinking about the establishment of one?

■ References

Adams M 1987 Deliveries – mothers or midwives – a study of communication styles in midwifery. MSc Dissertation (unpublished), University of Surrey

Alexander J 1984 Miscarriage: a cause for care. Primary Health Care   2 (10): 8–9

Bourne S, Lewis E 1984 Pregnancy after stillbirth or neonatal death: psychological risks and management. Lancet   ii: 31–3

Butler N 1969 Perinatal problems. Churchill Livingstone, Edinburgh

Butler N, Bonham A 1963 Perinatal mortality survey. Churchill Livingstone, Edinburgh

Culberg J 1972 Mental reactions of women to perinatal death in psychosomatic medicine. In Obstetrics and gynaecology: proceedings of the third international congress. Karger, Basel, London

Engel G 1962 Psychological disorders in health and disease. W B Saunders, Philadelphia

Forrest G C, Standish E, Baum J D 1982 Support after perinatal death: a study of support and counselling after perinatal bereavement. British Medical Journal   285: 1475–79

Gardner S, Morenstein G 1986 Perinatal grief and loss: an overview. Neonatal Network, October

Gibbons M 1984 Psychiatric sequelae of induced abortion. Journal of the Royal College of General Practitioners   34: 146–50

Giles P 1970 Reactions of women to perinatal death. Australia/New Zealand Journal of Obstetrics and Gynaecology   10: 207–10

Gohlish C 1985 Stillbirth. Midwife, Health Visitor and Community Nurse   21 (1): 12–16

Goodall J 1984 Notes for parents who have lost a child. Maternal and Child Health   1984 (April): 120–2

Health Education Bureau and SANDS A little lifetime. A booklet for parents whose babies have died around the time of birth. Health Education Bureau and SANDS, Ireland

Hill S 1989 Family. Michael Joseph, London

House of Commons Social Services Committee (HC) 1980 Report on perinatal and neonatal mortality (Short Report). HMSO, London

Hughes P 1987 The management of bereaved mothers: what is best? Midwives Chronicle 100 (1195): 226–29

Hutti M E 1988 A quick reference table of interventions to assist families to cope with pregnancy loss or neonatal death. Birth 15 (1): 33–5

Kennell J H, Slyter H, Klaus M 1970 The mourning response of parents to the death of a newborn infant. New England Journal of Medicine 283: 344–49

Kenyon S 1988 Support after termination for fetal abnormality. Midwives Chronicle 101 (1205): 190–91

Kohner N 1985 Midwives and stillbirth. RCM/HEC Workshop. RCM, London

Kubler-Ross E 1970 On death and dying. Tavistock Publications, London

Kumar R, Robson K 1978 Neurotic disturbance during pregnancy and the puerperium. In Sandler M (ed) Mental illness in pregnancy and the puerperium. Oxford University Press, Oxford

Lake M, Knuppel R, Murphy J, Johnson T 1983 The role of a grief support team following stillbirth. American Journal of Obstetrics and Gynecology 146 (8): 877–81

Lewis E, Bryan E M 1988 Management of perinatal loss of twins. British Medical Journal 297: 1321 (M) 1613 (C)

Lindman E 1944 Symptomatology and management of acute grief. American Journal of Psychiatry 101: 141–48

Maternity Services Advisory Committee 1985 Maternity care in action, Part III. Care of the mother and baby. HMSO, London

McMullan P 1986 Twin pregnancy. British Journal for Nurses in Child Health 1 (9): 264–65

Methven R C 1982 An examination of the process and content of the ante-natal booking interview. Unpublished MSc thesis, University of Manchester

Moore A 1987 Forgotten women. Midwives Chronicle 100 (1195): 242

Nash K 1987 It's still a baby. Midwives Chronicle 100 (1192): 123–25

Neustatter A, Newson G 1986 Mixed feelings: the experience of abortion. Pluto Press, London

Newman A 1984 Coping with grief. Nursing Times 81 (6): 32–4

Oakley A, McPherson A, Roberts H 1990 Miscarriage. Fontana, London

Office of Population Censuses and Surveys 1988 Birth statistics for England and Wales. OPCS, London

Parkes C M 1972 Bereavement: studies of grief in adult life. Penguin Books, Harmondsworth

Parkes C M 1980 Bereavement counselling: does it work? British Medical Journal 281: 3–6

Paykel E S, Emms E, Fletcher J, Rassaby E S 1980 Life events and social support in puerperal depression. British Journal of Psychiatry 136: 339–46

Penson J 1990 Bereavement – a guide for nurses. Harper and Row, London

Pepper L G, Knapp R J 1980 Motherhood and mourning. Praeger, New York

Roch S 1987 Sharing the grief. Nursing Times 83 (14): 52–3

Rice M 1982 Bereavement counselling: support available for the bereaved. Unpublished report of study leave. In RCM library
Tom-Johnson C 1990 Talking through grief. Nursing Times 86 (1): 44
Tschudin V 1987 Counselling skills for nurses (2nd ed). Baillière Tindall, London
United Kingdom Central Council 1989 A Midwife's Code of Practice for midwives practising in the United Kingdom, 2nd ed. UKCC, London
Webb C 1985a Barriers to sympathy. Nursing Mirror 160 (1): 5–7
Webb C 1985b Nurses' attitudes to therapeutic abortion. Nursing Times 81 (1): 44–7
White M P, Reynolds B, Evans T T 1984 Handling of death in special care nurseries and parental grief. British Medical Journal 289: 167–9

■ Suggested further reading

Beckey R D, Price R A, Okerson M, Riley K W 1985 Development of a perinatal grief checklist. Journal of Obstetric, Gynecologic and Neonatal Nursing 1985 14 (3): 194–99
David D L, Stewart M, Harmon R J 1988 Perinatal loss: providing emotional support for bereaved parents. Birth 15 (4): 242–46
Gardner S L, Morenstein G B 1986 Perinatal grief and loss: an overview. Neonatal Network 5 (2): 7–15
Health Education Bureau and SANDS A little lifetime. A booklet for parents whose babies have died around the time of birth. Health Education Bureau and SANDS, Ireland
Jolly J 1988 Missed beginnings. Austen Cornish for the Lisa Sainsbury Trust, London
Kubler-Ross E 1970 On death and dying. Tavistock Publications, London
Lewis E, Bryan E 1988 Management of perinatal loss of twins. British Medical Journal 297: 1321 (M) 1613 (C)
Oakley A, McPherson A, Roberts H 1984 Miscarriage. Fontana, London
Parkes C M 1972 Bereavement: studies of grief in adult life. Penguin Books, Harmondsworth
Penson J 1990 Bereavement: a guide for nurses: Chapter 6. Harper and Row, London
Rice M 1982 Bereavement counselling: support available for the bereaved. Unpublished report of study leave. In RCM library
Roch S 1987 Sharing the grief. Nursing Times 83 (14): 52–3
Speck P 1978 Loss and grief in medicine. Baillière Tindall, London
Tickner V J 1989 Counselling skills in midwifery practice. In Bennett V R, Brown L K (eds) Myles textbook for midwives (11th ed). Churchill Livingstone, Edinburgh
Tschudin V 1987 Counselling skills for nurses (2nd ed). Baillière Tindall, London
Walker C 1982 Attitudes to death and bereavement among cultural minority groups. Nursing Times 78 (50): 2106–09

■ Useful addresses

Foundation for the Study of Infant Deaths
(cot death research and support)
15 Belgrave Square
London SW1X 8PS
071 235 1721

Miscarriage Association
PO Box 24
Osset
West Yorks
WF5 9XG
0924 830515

National Childbirth Trust
Alexandra House
Oldham Terrace
Acton
London W3 6NH
081 992 8637

SAFTA (support after termination for fetal abnormality)
29–30 Soho Square
London W1V 6JB
071 439 6124

SANDS (Stillbirth and neonatal death society)
28 Portland Place
London W1 4DE
071 436 5881

TAMBA (Twins and multiple births association)
41 Fortuna Way
Aylesbury Park
Grimsby
South Humberside

Chapter 8

Teenage mothers

Marianne Mills

Pregnancy occurring in the teenage years is not a new phenomenon, nor are such pregnancies confined to any one country. In some cultures, indeed, girls may be given in marriage and become pregnant at a very early age. The author's enquiries at the Department of Anthropology, Glasgow University, suggested this to be particularly common practice in Tanzania, Kenya and Bangladesh. In these countries, the extended family is the usual unit and the young mother will receive support from the older members of the family.

The word 'teenage' covers a period of eight years and an enormous variety of circumstance and experience. Before considering pregnancy within this period it may be helpful to identify certain sub-groups, for example:

- The very young teenager, under 16;

- The older teenager aged 16–19;

- The unsupported teenager;

- The teenager supported by partner and family.

The teenage years provide a period of transition between childhood and adulthood when the 'developmental tasks of adolescence' (LaBarre 1969) are faced. Self identity is established, sets of values and ideals are formed by which to live and steps are taken towards independence. Sexual awareness develops during this period and sexual relationships may be entered into.

Levels of sexual activity vary amongst individuals. One young girl of 13 may be more sexually active than another aged 19. Rates of maturity also differ and some 13 years olds may be more or less mature (either physically or emotionally) than other individuals of 18 or 19.

The late teenage years may be a good time for pregnancy in a healthy young woman who is well supported by her partner and family. The situation is entirely different for the younger teenager and this chapter will therefore concentrate on the effects of pregnancy in this earlier age group; particular influences which affect these girls' perceptions of pregnancy are discussed. The physical and socioeconomic risks of early teenage pregnancy are explored as are the teenagers' own attitudes to pregnancy and the options open to them.

■ It is assumed that you are already aware of the following:

● The aetiology and implications of complications of pregnancy such as anaemia, pre-eclampsia, and preterm labour – as these may be more common in younger mothers (Duenholter *et al* 1975; Elliott & Beazley 1980; Osbourne *et al* 1981);

● The range of social, cultural and economic backgrounds from which clients in your unit's catchment area may come;

● The approximate ratio of teenage mothers and mothers aged 20 or over in your area; also what proportion, on average, of the teenagers are unsupported.

■ Social factors and teenage pregnancy

The occurrence of teenage pregnancy varies according to the girl's level of knowledge about contraception (Bury 1984). The outcome of teenage pregnancy is not always a viable infant due to the possibility of spontaneous or therapeutic abortion.

Throughout the world there is considerable variation in teenage pregnancy rates. In the USA it is estimated that one woman in ten aged between 15 and 19 becomes pregnant (Nadelson *et al* 1980). One fifth of all births are to women under 20 and one third of these are illegitimate. Nadelson's figures exclude women of 14 and under and it must be remembered that pregnancy does not always result in the birth of a viable child. In Great Britain the Registrar General publishes comprehensive data of birth and termination of pregnancy rates associated with particular age groups (the number of pregnancies ending in spontaneous abortion is not recorded). There has been a slight variation both in birth and abortion rates in the UK over recent years. Bury (1984) suggests that, although teenagers in Britain are less likely to become pregnant than in the late 1960s and early 1970s, one woman in five still becomes pregnant before she reaches the age of 20; four-fifths of these pregnancies are conceived outside marriage and approximately one-third end in termination. Government statistics (OPCS 1989) suggest that the termination of pregnancy rate for the 16–19 years age group is almost twice that for the population as a whole (see Fig. 8.1).

Figure 8.1 Abortion statistics for England and Wales, 1988

All ages:	13.22 per 1000 women
Under 16 years:	5.61 per 1000 women
16–19 years:	25.59 per 1000 women

Source: OPCS 1989

Several factors may contribute to a high teenage pregnancy rate. Peer pressure is very strong and some girls may consent to sexual intercourse because it is forbidden, uncharted territory which their friends (often untruthfully) say they have explored (Miles 1979). Sexual activity may be perceived as adult and exciting, like smoking or drinking. This perception is encouraged by the media through teen magazines or the behaviour of soap opera characters for example (Jones *et al* 1985). Advertising and pop music also emphasise sexuality. A boyfriend may be seen as necessary for social acceptability and it has traditionally been assumed that these boys may demand sex from their girlfriends as a condition of continuing the relationship. To many girls, however, this blackmail is unacceptable. In a survey in Glasgow, of 350 non-pregnant teenage girls from a variety of socioeconomic backgrounds, Mills (1988) found that over 50 per cent said that they would not agree to sexual intercourse under these circumstances and, furthermore, doubted that they would find an early sexual experience rewarding. This supported the findings of an earlier study (Cvetkovic *et al* 1978).

Society's attitude towards premarital sex has changed over the years and it would appear that pregnancy outside marriage is rarely condemned in the way it was 30 or 40 years ago. Many adults choose to live together outside marriage and teenage couples may follow suit enabled by greater financial independence among other factors.

Despite attempts by television programmes and magazine articles, the media seem to be less successful in educating young people about their bodies than in promoting the concept of romantic love (Jones *et al* 1985). Teenagers' knowledge of contraception techniques may be quite inadequate (Bury 1985). In a study of teenagers' understanding of birth control, Shah *et al* (1975) found that seven out of ten girls aged between 15 and 19 years did not think they could become pregnant. Other reasons for failing to use contraception ranged from perceived low risk because of age to wanting the pregnancy and a hedonistic objection to the precautions involved. Some teenagers may find the methods themselves unacceptable. Diaphragms and pessaries have been described as 'too messy' (Bury 1984) and providing a condom or taking the contraceptive pill may be seen to imply that, by anticipating the likelihood of sexual intercourse, the girl is 'promiscuous' (Bury 1984). It is possible, however, that the use of condoms will increase due to the fear of HIV infection.

Contraceptive advice and materials are readily available but used to a limited extent only by young couples. Nadelson *et al* (1980) found that although adolescent girls in their study had used some form of contraception, they had sometimes done so ineffectively or incorrectly and pregnancy had resulted. Very young girls are likely to know little about contraception; the topic may not have been discussed either at home or at school. Instead of factual and accurate knowledge, the girl may be influenced by beliefs that 'the Pill makes you fat' or that contraception is not available to those under 16, or she may be concerned that her parents will be told if she seeks contraceptive advice (Coyne 1986). Myths abound but from the variety of responses received by Nadelson and colleagues in their (1980) survey, the most common reflected a failure to acknowledge the consequences of sexual activity. Many teenage couples may be knowledgeable about contraception but ambivalent about its use, believing that pregnancy will not happen to them (Coyne 1986) or, if it does, that any ensuing problems will be solved by marriage (Nadelson *et al* 1980).

Teenage pregnancy is not always unplanned. Some girls may see pregnancy as an escape from a violent or unhappy home where they have been unloved or abused. In their study of schoolgirls, Shaffer *et al* (1978) found that girls from poor backgrounds where there was overcrowding, discordant family relationships and one parent families were more likely to become pregnant.

In certain areas drug, alcohol and solvent abuse may be perceived by teenagers as a means of coping with their lives. In the case of a pregnant teenager, the associated hazards of poor nutrition, anaemia, fetal alcohol syndrome, hepatitis B and HIV infection are well known. For further information, the reader is referred to Moira Plant's chapter 'Maternal alcohol and tobacco use during pregnancy' in the volume in this series on Antenatal Care, and to the chapter by Carolyn Roth and Janette Brierley, 'HIV infection – a midwifery perspective' in the volume in this series on Intrapartum Care. The book by Cameron (1988), cited in the 'Suggested further reading' list will also be useful.

Some teenagers may have left school lacking qualifications and with minimal prospects of obtaining employment. Society places much emphasis on achievement and unemployment may result in low self esteem (Shaffer *et al* 1978). Motherhood may be seen as the only worthwhile achievement possible; motherhood provides a 'job description' when no other job is available (Flett 1981). It has even been claimed (Daily Telegraph 1982) that some may become pregnant to increase their eligibility for council accommodation and increased state benefits. These views have been contested however (Gill 1989).

In her study of teenage girls in London, York and Liverpool, Clark (1989) found that 'they had got pregnant because of a complex variety of circumstances – just like women of any age'. Furthermore, while a recent survey (Mills 1988) provides anecdotal evidence from nonpregnant Glasgow

Figure 8.2 Benefits and resources available to teenage mothers

- At 1990/91 rates, a single mother aged between 16 and 18 will be eligible for:

Income support	£21.90
Dependent child under 11 allowance	£12.35
Family premium	£ 7.35
Lone parent allowance	£ 4.10

TOTAL: £45.70 per week

- A teenager who has been working or who has paid National Insurance stamps for a minimum of one year will, like other women, be entitled to Statutory Maternity Pay from her employer or Maternity Allowance from the DSS. Maternity Allowance as at 1st April 1990 is £35.70 per week for 18 weeks. She may also be entitled to a loan for specific purposes from the Social Fund

- Girls under the age of 16 are not entitled to Statutory Maternity Pay nor to Maternity Allowance as they have never been employed. Nor are they entitled to monetary benefits from the Social Fund

- A girl aged 15 or under is expected to live at home. If her parents are on a low income, they may be entitled to claim family credit as the qualifying income is based on the number of children in the household. Child benefit (£7.25 per week in 1990) for the girl herself will be paid to her parents until she leaves school, and they will also be able to claim child benefit for the baby

- Other non-monetary benefits, such as free prescriptions, free dental care and half fares on public transport, apply to all those under 16

- If parents are unable or unwilling to provide a home for a pregnant teenager or for a teenager and her baby, it is the responsibility of the Social Services to place girls aged under 16 years in care. For those over 16 years, a range of accommodation is provided by local authorities and housing trusts. Much of this is totally unsuitable for such a vulnerable group of young people

(This information has been compiled from Clark 1989, DSS 1990a, DSS 1990b, and conversations with senior social workers in Glasgow and Oxford)

teenagers who confirmed that the possibility of council housing might affect their attitude towards continuing a pregnancy should one occur, such perceptions are rarely matched by reality; little money will be forthcoming (see Fig. 8.2). Council accommodation may be difficult to obtain (particularly with the reduction in local authority housing stock that has occurred over the last few years) and the problems of living in unsuitable housing are compounded by the needs of the child (Clark 1989).

In some instances, the baby's father may be in a position to provide financial help – indeed legislation to ensure this is currently at the discussion stage. In such circumstances, maintenance can be sought either through direct request to the father or through a solicitor. The DSS will pay maintenance to the mother and then try to recoup the money from the father. If, however, the father is himself a teenager, the chances of his having any real income are small. Furthermore some girls, especially those who are under age, do not seek maintenance at all for fear of prosecution of the partner.

The outlook for girls under 16 is especially bleak as far as benefits are concerned. It is expected that they will be supported by their parents who receive child benefit for them. If they are in residential care they receive a pocket money allowance only. If they are runaways, they have to fend as best they can. It would seem certain, therefore, that as Coyne (1986) suggested, pregnancy does not only fail to improve the socioeconomic state of the teenager but, where there is no other support, the outlook for such mothers and their babies is worrying indeed.

Physical and mental health problems increase and so do stress levels. A number of studies (Smith *et al* 1973; Rutter & Madge 1976; Kempe & Kempe 1978; Shaffer *et al* 1978) suggest a correlation between unsuitable living conditions and child abuse. In a study of 214 parents of battered babies, Smith *et al* (1973) found that they were young and predominantly from poor socioeconomic backgrounds, that 76 per cent of the mothers had personality disorders.

If a girl becomes pregnant in her early teens, it is likely that she will present very late for antenatal care (Simms & Smith 1984; Coyne 1986). The reasons for this may include guilt or fear (real or imagined) that her boyfriend may be prosecuted. The true legal position is as follows:

- It is an absolute offence for a man to have intercourse with a girl under 13 years of age;

- It is an offence for a man to have intercourse with a girl aged between 13 and 16 unless he either believes himself to be legally married to her or he is under 24, has not been charged with any similar offence in the past and believes the girl to be over 16.

Under the Sexual Offences Act (1956) and the Sexual Offences Act for Scotland (1976), a boy of 14 is not liable to prosecution, nor does a girl under 16 commit an offence by having intercourse.

■ Medical and obstetric risks to mother and baby

A pregnant teenager may present late for antenatal care if she does not realise she is pregnant. She may be ignorant of the signs of pregnancy or her menstrual cycle may not yet be established. As well as incurring any risks which may be associated with a lack of antenatal care, the teenager may also be at risk from a number of specific complications during her pregnancy or in the postnatal period. Elliott and Beazley (1980) reported a slight increase in the perinatal mortality and morbidity rates of the babies of adolescent mothers they studied; there was a 10 per cent incidence of babies weighing below 2.5 kg. The higher perinatal mortality rate associated with teenage pregnancy is supported by the work of other authors (Duenholter *et al* 1975; Wells 1983) and there is evidence that the perinatal mortality rate in the babies of schoolgirls is up to three times higher than in the babies of mothers in their 20s (Babson & Clark 1983). In their study of 715 teenage primigravidae, Osbourne *et al* (1981) found no evidence of increased preterm labour and perinatal mortality in the teenage groups as a whole, but there were significant differences in these factors when the sub-groups of married and unmarried teenagers were compared. There were 32.6 perinatal deaths per total 1000 births among the babies of single mothers compared with 9.1 perinatal deaths per total 1000 births among the babies of the married teenagers ($p < 0.05$). McIntosh (1984) considers that the increased incidence of perinatal mortality arises primarily from an increase in babies of low birthweight and quotes Lawrence and Merritt (1981) who suggest that 85 per cent of these babies are preterm and that the low birthweight is associated with low socioeconomic group, smoking, alcohol, drugs and inadequate antenatal care.

Meningomyelocele and hydrocephalus are also increased in this group although the overall incidence of lethal malformation is low (Butler *et al*1969).

□ Problems during pregnancy

In a study of pregnant girls under the age of 15, Duenholter *et al* (1975) found that 34 per cent developed pregnancy induced hypertension compared with 25 per cent in a matched group of older women. Five years later, Elliott and Beazley (1980) reviewed the outcome of 263 pregnancies of girls under 16. They found a pre-eclampsia rate of 11 per cent, a reduction from rates suggested by other workers in the 1960s. Elliott and Beazley put forward the theory that this reduction may have resulted from improved antenatal care and earlier attendance at antenatal clinics. Osbourne *et al* (1981) also reported a reduction in the incidence of pregnancy induced hypertension in the 715 teenage mothers in their study (especially in the unmarried teenagers); indeed there was a slightly higher rate among the 464 women aged between 20 and 24 also included in this study.

Iron-deficiency anaemia is a commonly quoted complication of teenage pregnancy (Underhill & Atkins 1978). Fogel (1984) comments that poor dietary habits are common with adolescents. Fad diets are not unusual and nutritional know-how may be minimal. Moreover, a teenage girl may need to draw upon her nutritional resources for a spurt in her own growth as well as the growth of her baby. Osbourne *et al* (1981) found a highly significant increase of anaemia among pregnant teenagers (11 per cent compared to 5 per cent in the 20–24 year old age group – a p value of <0.001). They ascribe this partly to the later gestational age at booking and the consequent reduction in prophylactic iron tablets taken by these girls. Elliott and Beazley (1980) report an overall incidence of 11.5 per cent of anaemia (haemoglobin of less than 10 g/dl at some time during pregnancy) in their teenage mothers. In the group of mothers from a socially deprived background, the incidence of anaemia was three times as high as among those from a less deprived area (18 per cent as opposed to 6 per cent).

☐ **Problems during labour**

Elliott and Beazley (1980) found that labour was uncomplicated in the majority of teenagers and that the caesarean section rate in the young girls they studied was similar to the overall caesarean section rate for the hospital. Osbourne and colleagues (1981) found that labour was induced in 29.5 per cent of the teenagers but in a significantly higher number (36 per cent) of the women in their early 20s ($p < 0.05$). There was a corresponding difference in the occurrence of spontaneous labour ($p < 0.05$) with 58 per cent of the teenagers labouring spontaneously compared with 47.4 per cent of the older group. Significantly more of the teenagers had spontaneous vaginal deliveries ($p < 0.01$) and the casesarean section rate was also lower.

■ **Courses of action**

The very young mother is likely to have many psychological problems to address (Shaffer *et al* 1978). Her probable lack of maturity and emotional instability may lead to child neglect or abuse through frustration, depression or a sense of isolation if she has inadequate social, emotional or financial support (Smith *et al* 1973). In extreme cases the baby may even be abandoned in the way that hits newspaper headlines from time to time.

A teenager's parents may perceive her pregnancy as a betrayal not only of their plans for her future but also of themselves and the rest of the family. Such feelings may lead them to reject or isolate her (Miles 1979).

Changes in society's attitude affect the decisions made by the mother which, without adequate counselling, may not be decisions which will improve her quality of life or that of her child (Shaffer *et al* 1978; Black 1986).

Termination of pregnancy is likely to be seen as an option unless the pregnancy is not acknowledged until it is too far advanced. In 1988, the number of terminations carried out on women resident in Great Britain rose to 180 000. One quarter of these were carried out on girls aged under 20 (41 000 for the 16–19 age group and 4000 on the under 16s) compared with just over one fifth in 1971 (Central Statistics Office 1990). (See also Fig. 8.1 on page 127 above.)

The 350 girls interviewed in the Glasgow survey (Mills 1988) were, however, largely against abortion. They commented that abortion equated with murder, that the baby had a right to life even if it were handicapped, and that the mother should take full responsiblity for her actions. Some condoned abortion in cases of rape, incest or child abuse or when the mother was very young indeed. These girls were not, to the best of the researcher's knowledge, pregnant at the time of the survey, nor had they been pregnant. It is, of course, possible that their opinions would change if they were to become pregnant.

Adoption is another course of action that may be considered but it is often fraught with practical and emotional difficulties. The mother may feel guilty at the prospect of giving her baby up for adoption and may, later, spend years wondering whether he is happy or whether he would understand why she had appeared to abandon him. Furthermore the mother has the right to change her mind up until such time as the adoption has been granted by the courts – an unsettling and potentially distressing state of affairs not only for her but also for the adoptive parents who may have been waiting for years for a baby they can call their own and who must have cared for the child for at least three months before the court hearings.

While acknowledging feelings of guilt and loss, some girls nevertheless wish to proceed with adoption believing that they are giving their baby the best chance of a happy life. Adoption can also be seen as providing an opportunity for a fresh start on the part of the teenager herself. Midwives should be alert for the 'empty arm syndrome' (Miles 1979) however; feelings of grief for the 'lost' baby, possibly compounded by guilt, may lead the girl to embark on another pregnancy when she does not have any more resources than she had before. Many mothers whose babies are stillborn obtain some ease from holding the dead baby (see the chapter in this volume by Margaret Adams and Joyce Prince, 'Care of the grieving parent with special reference to stillbirth'); the same may also apply for a mother about to give up her living baby. It may not, therefore, always be advisable to agree without further counselling or discussion to a girl's request that the baby be placed out of her sight and hearing as soon as it is born.

In situations where termination or adoption are considered, expert counselling should be given to help pregnant girls and their families to make, and learn to live with, the decisions that are right for them. The issues and techniques involved in this aspect of care are too important to be included in a chapter of this size but the reader might find the two items on counselling skills (Tschudin 1987; Tickner 1989) cited in the 'Suggested further reading' list useful.

A teenage mother may decide to keep her baby and if she does, less stigma will be attached to her situation by society at large than she would have encountered a generation ago. Some help will usually be available, if it is required, for those on low incomes from the local authority and the Department of Social Security (see Fig 8.2 on page 129 above). Girls under the age of 16 are considered to be the responsibility of either their parents or the Social Services Department.

Ideally the DSS leaflet FB8, 'Babies and Benefits', should be made available at antenatal and postnatal clinics. It may also be helpful if midwives having contact with teenage girls are able to give them the address, telephone number and opening hours for the nearest Citizens' Advice Bureau who will be able to give full details of the latest information on benefits, housing and other entitlements.

The girl's family may accept her pregnancy without too much ado; indeed, the idea of a forthcoming baby may be welcomed actively by its prospective grandparents whose own children are growing up and who may miss having a baby to care for. In such cases, the baby may be assimilated into the family with ease. Problems may arise, however, if the baby is brought up by its grandparents as if it were the brother or sister of its natural mother, or if the grandmother attempts to dictate to her daughter about child rearing.

If the teenager is old enough, and her relationship with the baby's father is sufficiently stable, marriage or cohabitation may be seen as a means of providing social, emotional and financial support. This solution may, however, bring its own problems; Leete's (1975) study of population trends suggested that teenage marriages were more likely to end in divorce than those where both partners had married at a later age. In a study of 533 teenage mothers, Simms and Smith (1983) found that of the 328 who married, 16 had separated and at least eight had been physically abused by their husbands within 18 months of marriage. Isolation (particularly if the marriage was not approved of by the young people's parents), poverty, immaturity and inexperience of dealing with the realities of parenthood may all be contributing factors in the breakdown of relationships. Figures for 1980–84 produced by OPCS (1986) indicate that 10 per cent of women who married between the ages of 16 and 19 were separated within two years and 3 per cent were divorced. This compares with a separation rate of 7 per cent in two years among women married between the ages of 20 and 24 and 8 per cent in two years among women married between the ages of 25 and 29. The divorce rate for the same period among women in these older groups was, however, comparable to that of the teenagers at 2–3 per cent.

Opinions vary about the advisability of the very young mother looking after her baby on her own. Certainly the child should remain with its natural parents wherever possible (Miles 1979). In some cases, however, if the couple are very young and immature, are poorly educated and have a reduced chance of employment, the outlook for the family is bleak. Such circumstances are potentially hazardous for a child (Smith *et al* 1973).

☐ Opportunities for mothers

When pregnancy occurs in the early teenage years, the girl's education will inevitably suffer some disruption. This may well have more far reaching effects on her chances of higher education or employment. Both this disruption and an existing state of social or economic deprivation can narrow the mother's horizons and thereby increase the risk of her baby growing up to be a poor achiever (Shaffer *et al* 1978). So the cycle of deprivation continues (Rutter & Madge 1976).

One American study (Klerman & Jekel 1973) indicated that a return to education was more influential in preventing further pregnancies than the provision of contraceptives. If a girl receives adequate support, especially from her own family, she may be encouraged to continue her own education and to help her child to develop his potential.

In theory, home tuition is available for all girls not attending school during pregnancy and for a short time after the baby's birth. The actual provision, however, varies with individual education authorities (Miles 1979). In San José, California, there is a high school which makes special provision for pregnant schoolgirls and provides a crèche for schoolgirl mothers (Clare 1986). This example has been followed in Britain by the Avon Health Authority (Thomas, personal communication) but such initiatives are far from widespread and may be fraught with problems. Schools may fear for their reputations if they are seen to be accepting pregnancy among their students and the cost of establishing a crèche may be too great for any one school. Teachers would certainly need to be sensitive and flexible as a new mother might find it difficult to do the same amount of work soon after giving birth as she did before.

☐ Parenthood education

Paradoxically, pregnant teenagers are often in great need of parentcraft education but, for a variety of reasons, are often reluctant to attend 'normal' parentcraft sessions (Simms & Smith 1984; Coyne 1986). Schemes have, therefore, been set up by midwives and others, enabling pregnant teenagers to meet as a group accompanied by friends or partners (Evans & Parker 1985; Nunnerley 1985; Todd *et al* 1988). A midwife who organises and teaches these groups needs to be approachable, sympathetic, sensitive, knowledgeable and skilled at counselling (Evans & Parker 1985). She may have to face some difficult challenges – for example a girl who is deaf, who is addicted to drugs, or whose intelligence is low – so she will need to be both innovative and highly committed.

There are all too few antenatal groups in the UK catering for the special needs of teenagers (Bury 1984). They are not easy to set up and common problems encountered may involve accommodation and recruitment (Minns 1989; Watson 1989). Attendance may be poor, although Coyne (1986) found that where antenatal education was specifically geared towards teenagers, both attendance and motivation to learn improved. It may be considered, however, that the number of pregnant teenagers in any particular area is too few to make the running of a special course of classes worthwhile and girls in this age group are unlikely to be able to afford, or to be motivated towards, travelling long distances.

It is helpful if teenage groups can continue to meet postnatally, thus providing a venue for young mothers to meet for company and mutual support (Minns 1990). The full implications of motherhood are rarely realised until this time. Pregnancy can be an 'unreal' state in which the girl is the centre of attention, reality registering only when the baby actually arrives and, even more so, when she takes it home. The girl may then experience loneliness, depression and frustration. She will be in considerable need of professional and family support, as well as the support of her peers (Miles 1979).

Attendance at parentcraft classes does not necessarily prepare any mother fully for her first child. Many mothers forget what they have learned several weeks earlier and need reminding; this need is likely to be increased in very young mothers. Teaching on a one to one basis may be required but there are obvious social advantages to teaching teenagers in postnatal groups. Such classes could cover topics as diverse as health education (including contraception), homemaking, cookery and the principles of good nutrition, managing a limited budget and advice on claiming income support and other benefits. Unfortunately few such groups exist at present, though the 'Teenage club' at the Royal Berkshire (Todd et al 1988) actively encourages postnatal attenders and postnatal reunions were organised formally for the teenage antenatal groups from Kings College Hospital (Nunnerley 1985). There is, however, enormous scope throughout the country for the implementation of more schemes (Watson 1989; Minns 1989, 1990). Similarly a European Collaborative Committee for Child Health (Wells 1983) recommends that more opportunities be made available for young mothers to learn basic mothering skills.

In some areas there are flats (perhaps provided by the Social Services Department) to which young, single mothers may go to learn homemaking skills. One such unit in Glasgow is run as a day centre (Long 1989) and another (also in Glasgow) as a teaching tenancy for those who are setting up home for the first time and who are in need of support and education, for example young mothers who have been in care until this point in their lives (Glass 1989).

☐ Health education in schools

For many reasons, some of which have already been discussed, the early teenage years are not good years in which to embark on pregnancy. Human nature being what it is, however, many teenagers will become sexually active and pregnancy will occur for some of them (Jordan & Skuse 1987). Women, including young teenage women, should be encouraged to make their own decisions about their life and future. Health education is vital to enable them to make such decisions as whether to take part in or refrain from sexual intercourse. Assertiveness skills may also be developed to help ensure that if a girl would rather not take part in sexual activity, she feels able to refuse.

The standard of health education in schools varies. Although the girls in Mills' (1988) survey were from six different schools, most of them felt that they had had little sex education beyond Section 6 of the biology module (Scotland) and a visit by a representative from a firm manufacturing tampons.

Health visitors carry the responsibility for health education in many schools and many of their programmes are excellent. All too often, however, health education (and in particular sex education) falls to whichever teacher has time to undertake it. This author feels strongly that the subject is far too important to be approached in such a haphazard fashion. Rather, it should be undertaken as a properly thought out and planned programme by a team of specialists in the field of health education. Such a team could comprise health visitors, nurses, midwives, doctors and others outside the health professions, especially parents.

A suggested outline for a health education programme, to be taught to boys as well as girls, is set out in Fig. 8.3. Schemes such as this may already exist in some schools, especially in the United States (Keenan 1986), but they are not widely available in Great Britain.

Pregnancy during the teenage years is inevitable as these are the years of learning and experimentation. With a better example from their parents, more thorough health education programmes and fewer 'mixed messages' from the media, youngsters may become more aware of the consequences of their actions and the numbers of unwanted pregnancies reduced. The Trust for the Study of Adolescence has produced two booklet/cassette packages (Coleman 1989a; 1989b) specifically to help the parents of teenagers. In schools, much more emphasis should be put on teaching about contraception and interpersonal skills, as well as on encouraging discussion of moral issues and questions of responsibilities.

Figure 8.3 Suggested outline for a health education programme for schools

Kindergarten/Infant school	Simple principles of health and hygiene set out in reading primer
Junior/primary school	The functions of different systems of the body, principles of caring for one's body. In the final year, the reproductive system
High school/secondary school	The reproductive system in more detail and related to puberty; this should be accompanied by open and frank discussion about puberty, emotions and the problems and pleasures of growing up. By age 15–16, such discussions would centre upon human relationships – loving and caring, respect and trust, the desirability of a stable relationship before undertaking the responsibility of creating another human life, contraception, pregnancy, the problems of parenthood (especially single parenthood), sexually transmitted diseases and the dangers of substance abuse.
	Parallel studies of religious and moral philosophy, as well as home making and budgetting skills, may also be instituted by the appropriate teaching departments

■ Recommendations for clinical practice in the light of currently available evidence

1. Midwives should foster links with local schools in order to encourage adequate teaching on interpersonal relationships, contraception, and responsible sexual behaviour as well as realistic preparation for family life.

2. Midwives should foster links with local education authorities to encourage the setting up of schemes that enable pregnant schoolgirls to continue their education.

3. Midwives should be aware of the health education material produced for young people, as well as that produced for the parents of teenagers by the Trust for the Study of Adolescence.

4. There should be more widespread advertising of family planning clinics.

5. Individualised antenatal care should be given to pregnant teenagers. Where possible, they should see the same midwife every time and parentcraft teaching should be emphasised. Special courses of antenatal classes for this age group should be developed wherever possible.

6. Postnatal care should be given for as long as is necessary and where possible should be combined with regular visits from the health visitor and/or the social worker. Support groups should be set up and encouraged.

7. At a national level, midwives could lobby for better housing provision and adequate benefits for single, unsupported teenage mothers.

■ Practice check

● Do you know the teenage pregnancy rate in your area? Do you consider that your health authority makes proper provision to address the needs of teenage mothers?

● Do you have a structured health education programme to offer to schools?

● What health education material do you have available or accessible to recommend to teenagers themselves, or to their parents?

● Does your authority have a separate antenatal clinic for teenage mothers and provide parenthood education for them suited to their needs?

● Is any follow-up support available for these teenage mothers and their babies? If not, do you know where to refer the mother?

□ Acknowledgements

Thanks are due to Valerie Levy from the Royal Cornwall Hospital, Truro, and to Helen Minns from the John Radcliffe Hospital, Oxford, for their advice and suggestions and to Richenda Milton-Thompson for her help in improving the structure of my text.

This article reflects the personal opinion of the author and does not necessarily represent the views of the Greater Glasgow Health Board.

■ References

Babson S G, Clarke N G 1983 Relationships between infant death and maternal age. Journal of Paediatrics   103: 391–3
Black D 1986 Schoolgirl mothers. British Medical Journal   293: 1047

Bury J K 1984 Teenage pregnancy in Britain. Birth Control Trust, London

Bury J K 1985 Teenage pregnancy. British Journal of Obstetrics and Gynaecology 92: 1081–83

Butler N R, Alberman E D, Schatt 1969 The congenital malformations. In Butler N R, Alberman E D (eds) Perinatal problems. Livingstone, Edinburgh

Central Statistics Office 1990 Social Trends 20. HMSO, London

Clare A 1986 Lovelaw: 16–17. BBC Publications, London

Clark E 1989 Young single mothers today: a qualitative study of housing and support needs. National Council for One Parent Families, London

Coleman J 1989a Teenagers in the family. Trust for the Study of Adolescence, Brighton

Coleman J 1989b Teenagers under stress. Trust for the Study of Adolescence, Brighton

Coyne A-M 1986 Schoolgirl mothers. HEC Research Report 2. Health Education Council, London

Cvetkovic G, Grote B, Lieberman E J, Miller W 1978 Sex role development, teenage fertility related. Adolescence 13: 231–36

Daily Telegraph 1982 'Getting pregnant to beat the dole' claim. 30th December

Department of Social Security 1990a Babies and benefits. Leaflet FB 8. HMSO, London

Department of Social Security 1990b Leaflet SB 20. HMSO, London

Duenholter J H, Jiminez J M, Baumann G 1975 Pregnancy performance of patients under fifteen years of age. Obstetrics and Gynecology 46: 49–52

Elliott H R, Beazley J M 1980 A clinical study of pregnancy in younger teenagers in Liverpool. Journal of Obstetrics and Gynaecology 1 (1): 16–19

Evans G, Parker P 1985 Preparing teenagers for pregnancy. Midwives Chronicle 98 (1172): 239–40

Flett U 1981 Teenage sexuality – a dilemma for all generations. Times Educational Supplement, 13th November

Fogel C I 1984 The adolescent mother: special problems. In Houston M J (ed) Maternal and infant health care. Recent Advances in Nursing 9. Churchill Livingstone, Edinburgh

Gill L 1989 A teenage myth? The Times, 29th September

Glass B 1989 Development of the Walpole Housing Association. Journal of the Special Housing Association 9 (Jan/Feb): 18–19

Jones E F, Forrest J D, Goldman N, Henshaw S K, Lincoln R, Rossoff J I, Westoff C F, Wulf D 1985 Determinants and policy implications: teenage pregnancy in developed countries. Alan Guttmacher Institute, New York

Jordan T, Skuse P 1987 Adolescent understanding of child development. Maternal and Child Health 1987 (11): 326–29

Keenan T 1986 School based adolescent health care program. Pediatric Nursing 12 (5): 365–69

Kempe R S, Kempe C H 1978 The abusive parent. In Bruner J, Cole M, Lloyd B (eds) Child abuse. Fontana/Open Books Original, London

Klerman L V, Jekel J F 1973 School age mothers: problems, programs and policy. Shoestring Press, Connecticut

LaBarre M 1969 The triple crisis: adolescence, early marriage and parenthood. Part 1 Motherhood, the double jeopardy, the triple crisis, illegitimacy today. National Council of Illegitimacy, New York

Lawrence R A, Merritt T A 1981 Infants of adolescent mothers: perinatal, neonatal and infancy outcome. Seminars in Perinatology 5: 19–32

Leete R 1975 Marriage, divorce. Population Trends 3: 3–8

Long R 1989 Life on the breadline. Glasgow Evening Times, 14th February

McIntosh N 1984 Baby of a schoolgirl. Archives of Diseases in Childhood 59: 915–17

Miles M 1979 Pregnant at school. Joint working party on pregnant schoolgirls and schoolgirl mothers. National Council for One Parent Families, London

Mills M J G 1988 Teenage attitudes to pregnancy in Glasgow. Midwives Chronicle 101 (1207): 243–45

Minns H R 1989 Young mums' club. Nursing Times 85 (28): 68–69

Minns H R 1990 Infant feeding in adversity 1: Young mothers. Midwives Chronicle 103 (1224): 3–4

Nadelson C C, Notman M T, Gillon J 1980 Sexual knowledge and attitudes of adolescents: relationship to contraceptive use. Obstetrics and Gynecology 55: 340–45

Nunnerley R 1985 Teenage dilemma. Midwives Chronicle 98 (1172): 244–48

Office of Population Censuses and Surveys 1986 Divorce statistics for England and Wales 1980–1984. OPCS, London

Office of Population Censuses and Surveys 1989 Abortion statistics for England and Wales 1988. OPCS, London

Osbourne G K, Howat R C L, Jordan M M 1981 The obstetric outcome of teenage pregnancy. British Journal of Obstetrics and Gynaecology 88: 215–21

Rutter M, Made N 1976 Cycles of disadvantage. Heinemann, London

Shaffer D, Pettigrew A, Wolkind S, Zajicek E 1978 Psychiatric aspects of pregnancy in schoolgirls: a review. Psychological Medicine 8: 119–29

Shah F, Zelnik M, Kantner J F 1975 Unprotected intercourse among unwed teenagers. Family Planning Perspective 7: 39–44

Simms M, Smith S 1983 Teenage mothers and their partners: a survey in England and Wales. DHSS Research Report 15. HMSO, London

Simms M, Smith S 1984 Teenage mothers: late attenders at medical and antenatal care. Midwife, Health Visitor and Community Nurse 20: 192–200

Smith S, Hanson R, Noble S 1973 Parents of battered babies: a controlled study. British Medical Journal 17: 388–91

Todd J E, Lapthorn J, McIntosh J 1988 Teenage club at the Royal Berkshire. Midwives Chronicle 101 (1207): 238–40

Underhill R, Atkins N 1978 Schoolgirl pregnancies. Journal of Maternal and Child Health 3: 404–09

Watson G 1989 Births to 16 year olds and under. Association of Radical Midwives Magazine 42 (Autumn): 20

Wells N 1983 Teenage mothers. European Collaborative Committee for Child Health. Children's Research Fund, Liverpool

■ Suggested further reading

Cameron J S 1988 Solvent abuse: a guide for the carer. Croom Helm, London

Clark E 1989 Young single mothers today: a qualitative study of housing and support needs. National Council for One Parent Families, London

Coleman J 1989 Teenagers in the family. 72 page booklet and 60 minute cassette for parents. Trust for the Study of Adolescence, 23 New Road, Brighton

Coleman J 1989 Teenagers under stress. 56 page booklet and 60 minute cassette for parents. Trust for the Study of Adolescence, 23 New Road, Brighton

Kuczynski H J 1988 An approach to preventing adolescent pregnancy. Midwives Chronicle   101 (1207): 234–37

Minns H R 1990 Infant feeding in adversity 1: young mothers. Midwives Chronicle   103 (1224): 3–4

Tickner V J 1989 Counselling skills in midwifery practice. In Bennett V R, Brown L K (eds) Myles textbook for midwives (11th ed). Churchill Livingstone, Edinburgh

Todd J E, Lapthorn J, McIntosh J 1988 Teenage club at Royal Berkshire. Midwives Chronicle   101 (1207): 238–40

Tschudin V 1987 Counselling skills for nurses (2nd ed). Baillière Tindall, London

Watson G 1989 Births to 16 year olds and under. Association of Radical Midwives Magazine   42 (Autumn): 20

Chapter 9

Quality assurance in postnatal care

Rowan Nunnerley

This chapter considers the concept of quality assurance and its relation to postnatal care. It will consider the theory related to quality assurance and select some of the measurement tools which are available: questionnaires, peer observation surveys and suggestion boxes. Quality circles can identify areas which require improvement and if readers are familiar with Monitor or performance indicators, for example, they may want to consider specific applications of these to the midwifery setting.

Postnatal care is a vital part of the child rearing process but, unfortunately, it has been given a low priority in many maternity units. 'In the past, inadequate and unqualified care has resulted in poor communications, conflicting advice, confusion and a marring of the mother's joy and satisfaction' (Samuel & Balch 1985).

The UKCC (1986) Midwives' Rules state that a midwife has to provide postnatal care to the mother and her baby for a period of not less than 10 days and not more than 28 days after the end of labour. Postnatal care should include consideration of the following topics:

- The physical health and wellbeing of the mother;

- The psychological and emotional responses of the mother to parenthood and her reactions to her child;

- The emotional health of the family unit;

- The amount, the type and the quality of the social support that the family unit is receiving.

There are huge psychological, physical and social adjustments that motherhood can demand of new, often inexperienced mothers and it is ironic that postnatal care has been the facet of maternity services least well supported by management, medical staff and even midwives. One hopes that this is a situation which is less likely to arise in maternity units today (Ray 1986). It is important, however, to examine midwifery practice, criticise the way postnatal care is delivered and make systematic efforts to improve the quality of care.

The assurance of quality requires agreed expectations (standards and objectives), comparisons (of actual practice against expectations) and effective action, to reconcile the two. Quality assurance can be defined as 'a commitment to excellence in the delivery of care and a professional accountability for the care given' (Nursing Standard 1987).

Over the past five years, there have been changes in midwifery practice which, undoubtedly, have influenced the quality of postnatal care and have been implemented to improve client satisfaction and job satisfaction for the midwife. The introduction of the midwifery process has taken place in many units. Individualised care plans have been designed for mothers and babies which should enable client participation and continuity of midwifery care. Linking in with continuity of care is the concept of team midwifery. This increases the likelihood of care being given by the same midwife, or by a small group of two or three midwives thus increasing client satisfaction.

In order to meet individual client's needs, a more flexible day routine now exists in most maternity units and the majority of women have a choice as to how long they stay in hospital postnatally.

Parent education over the past years has changed for the better. A greater variety of teaching methods and audiovisual aids are now being used and there is recognition of the need to provide classes for different client groups (teenagers, ethnic minority groups, couples, and even adoptive parents). See also the chapter by Tricia Murphy-Black on 'Antenatal education' in the volume in this series on *Antenatal Care*.

■ It is assumed that you are already familiar with the following:

- The UKCC Midwives' Rules, Midwives' Code of Practice and the Code of Professional Conduct.

- The Maternity Services Advisory Committee reports, particularly Part III (1985) which concentrates on postnatal care.

- The numerous articles and publications on postnatal care, the quality of care and assessing quality, many of which can be found in any hospital library and it would be advisable to seek some of them out. A selection of such titles is included in the 'Further reading' list at the end of this chapter.

■ Theory related to quality assurance

In order to understand the subject of 'quality assurance', the reader will need to be familiar with the concepts of quality, quality assurance, standards and criteria. Some knowledge of the variety of measurement tools for assessing quality would also be helpful.

☐ Quality and quality assurance

Quality is said to have a degree or standard of excellence and is also the margin between desirability and reality (Nursing Standard 1987). Quality assurance is a process which can be directed towards evaluating the quality of care that is provided, through setting standards of care and implementing mechanisms for ensuring these standards are met. One such process has three components, as detailed below.

1. *A value system* – which determines the quality of care. In the NHS there are certain policies, procedures, statements of philosophy and job descriptions which exist. In addition, all midwives must abide by the UKCC (1986) Midwives' Rules and Code of Practice.

2. *An appraisal system* – being the collection of information about performance and the comparison of the fit between the performance and the standard that has been set.

3. *A response system.* When standards are met or improvement occurs, this constitutes progress and/or excellence. If standards are not met, immediate change may be necessary, perhaps in a policy or procedure.

☐ Standards

A standard is an accepted or approved example of something, against which others are judged or measured. A standard:

● Is a principle of priority;

● Has honesty and integrity;

● Is a level of excellence or quality of recognised authority;

● Can be laid down at a national, district or local level;

● Is a plain statement of performance (Dunne 1986).

Standards include care plans or formats and may cover such areas as manpower levels, equipment, clinical practice, midwifery education (ward learning climate) and clients' responses to care delivered.

Having agreed upon the standards, the next step is to measure present practice against the desired, pre-set standard to determine whether or not the service provided is acceptable or whether some form of remedial action and in-service education needs to be taken.

☐ **Criteria**

The basic standard can be broken down into a list of criteria, a criterion being a measurable aspect of desired performance (Kitson, unpublished). The criteria checklists are usually divided into three sections, as indicated below.

1. *Structure* – what should be provided in terms of the organisation and resources to meet the standard; this checklist should include staffing levels, skill mix, shift patterns, ward layout, admission policy and information training.

2. *Process*. What should the staff do to bring about the type of care outlined in the standard? Topics to be included in this checklist will be relationships with the client, items of nursing/midwifery care, information given.

3. *Outcome*. This covers the end result in terms of the client's health and satisfaction. What can be observed to prove that the standard of care has been met? Has the client's independence been improved, for example, or her anxiety reduced? Does she understand what is being done and why?

Standards and criteria should be Relevant, Understandable, Measureable, Behavioural and Achievable (RUMBA).

It is important to involve the staff in formulating standards for their own work area. Likewise the staff will need to assess and evaluate the situation to ascertain whether the quality of care has improved as a direct result of setting standards. This can be carried out by following some simple principles:

● Identify the required standards and criteria, using the checklists (structure, process and outcome) outlined above;

● Secure measurements for the standards so as to ascertain whether or not they are being maintained;

- Interpret the strengths and weaknesses of the particular area/organisation before taking action;

- The course of action will need to build upon the found strengths and minimise the discovered weaknesses;

- There may be several options to choose from but the most democratic form of action is to use a problem-solving approach;

- Once the action has been taken it will be essential to identify the values to the client, to the staff and to the organisation.

☐ Quality circles

Quality circles are full scale problem-solving groups. Not only do they identify what is wrong, they are also concerned with devising solutions and, with management approval, ensure implementation and monitoring of the results (Christie & O'Reilly 1984). Quality circles are an important element in a process whereby staff at every layer in an organisation work together as a team to improve the quality of service and working life. They involve everyone from the top to bottom of the organisation, open up new channels of communication, encourage team work and improve job satisfaction (Hyde 1984).

■ The problem-solving approach includes the following stages:

- Brainstorming for a likely problem;

- Selecting the most relevant problems;

- Analysis and investigation of the chosen problem;

- Finding a solution to the problem;

- Implementing the decision which has been taken by the manager responsible.

Quality circles which achieve goals and receive management support can encourage more quality circles to form and become self-perpetuating. Job satisfaction is likely to result as staff become involved with decision-making. Management and worker contribute together to provide a service of high quality to the customer.

■ Quality assurance in relation to postnatal care

Postnatal care should be given a high priority and a basic standard of service must be provided which will meet mothers' and babies' health needs as well as the families' wider social needs.

No single pattern of family life is likely to prevail into the 21st century and one standard pattern of service is not likely to meet all the needs. A range of options should be provided for different individuals and different communities. Parents' perceptions of the quality of their postnatal care is very important and it is not always related to the standards chiefly considered important by the professional.

☐ Practical application of the measurement tools: standards

The All Wales Planning Committee (1986) was one of the first bodies to write standards of care for midwifery. One such example is the safe and comfortable transfer of a mother from the delivery suite to the postnatal

Figure 9.1 Setting standards of care

Example:	Transfer of mother from delivery suite to postnatal ward
Aim:	The mother is admitted to a safe, welcoming environment
Role:	The midwife receives the mother and baby to the postnatal ward

ward (see Fig. 9.1). The midwifery actions required to perform this activity to the required standard would be:

- To make an assessment of the mother's and baby's physical condition;
- To instruct the mother about the nurse call system;
- To place the baby in a cot at the bedside;
- To invite the birth partner to join the mother if he is not already with her;
- To ensure that liquid refreshment is available and within easy reach;
- To record and assess intravenous therapy, epidurals and other treatments if in progress;
- To store the mother's property as agreed by the health authority's policy.

A second example might be concerned with food in the postnatal ward (Nunnerley 1988). The aim here would be to provide a diet which is nutritious, attractive and has suitable size portions, so as to enable a postnatal mother to recuperate. If she is breastfeeding her diet should enable her to provide an adequate milk supply for the baby.

The objectives in this context might be:

- To provide a suitable menu choice taking into account the specific requirements of mothers who are vegetarian, who belong to an ethnic minority group, or who have had a caesarean section;

- To have attractive, health enhancing food – such as wholemeal bread, fresh vegetables, fruit salad and more fibre content;

- To have a variety of meals including light snacks, fresh sandwiches, biscuits and cheese and fresh fruit;

- To provide a microwave in each ward so that food can be warmed up if a mother is feeding her baby at the time the meals are given out (this should be checked with the catering officer prior to installation);

- To have a suitable container to transport the food, with separate compartments for hot and cold food.

☐ **Practical application of the measurement tools: checklist of structure/ process/outcome**

A more formal approach using the criteria checklists, (covering structure, process and outcome), and based on Kitson's work, is shown in Fig. 9.2.

■ **Methods for assessing the quality for care applied to postnatal care in hospital**

Three methods for assessing the quality of postnatal care in hospital were carried out during a research project (Nunnerley 1988) and the chosen methods were, firstly, questionnaires (to mothers and staff); secondly, peer observation; and thirdly, a suggestion box. A brief resumé of the work carried out in this project is given below.

☐ **Survey/questionnaire**

Questionnaires (see appendix to this chapter) were designed for the postnatal mothers and the hospital staff so as to compare the results. Four

Figure 9.2   The three tier criteria checklist (structure, process, outcome)

Topic:	Independence and involvement
Sub topic:	Pre-induction of labour information giving
Care group:	Pregnant women undergoing induction of labour
Standard statement:	All expectant mothers will be provided with information giving the reasons for possible side effects/and outcomes of labour/delivery
Criteria:	**1.** *Structure* Written leaflets and information sheets on the reasons/methods for induction of labour to be provided
	2. *Process* The midwife will assess the mother's needs (and those of her partner) prior to and on admission so as to ensure relevant verbal, written and visual information is provided before induction of labour The midwife's assessment and actions are recorded in the client's care plan
	3. *Outcome* The mother is able to explain: (a) the reasons/methods for induction of labour (b) possible side effects and outcomes of labour/delivery (c) the midwife's care/observations during labour

district hospitals were chosen for the survey. These were all district general hospitals, but in different geographical locations. Each hospital was visited by the researcher who handed out the questionnaires in person to mothers and staff, then collected them later on the same day. This enabled an 85–90 per cent response rate. It also enabled any discrepancies and misunderstandings regarding the questionnaires to be clarified at the time – which proved invaluable when it came to revising for later work.

The questionnaire designed for mothers covered the following topics: type of delivery, previous children, arrival on the postnatal ward, daily care, pain relief, postnatal exercises, feeding the baby, linen, postnatal teaching and visiting hours. The staff questionnaire was concerned with ward profile, postnatal care, feeding advice, postnatal teaching, and with visiting hours.

☐ **Staff questionnaire (see pages 158–60)**

One interesting aspect which arose from the staff survey was that the hospital with the highest bed occupancy and the lowest staffing levels provided the highest quality of postnatal care. This could relate to the management and education of midwifery staff which have an impact on maintaining high standards. Whatever their circumstances, these staff were able to provide a high quality of care to the mothers.

☐ **Mothers' questionnaire (see pages 161–64)**

The main areas of concern highlighted by this survey involved the 'hotel services' (the quality of food, linen services and cleanliness).

Advice given to mothers regarding breastfeeding was often conflicting, partly because there were different staff looking after mothers and many of those were very temporary in nature, being hired from an agency. In the mothers' opinion agency staff appeared to provide poor quality care but generally the attitudes of all staff needed to change. A sensitive approach is required for each mother and in spite of business and shortage of staff, time should be made to listen and explain aspects of care to the mother and her partner.

☐ **Peer observation survey**

The idea of this peer observation survey originated from 'Qualpacs' (Quality Patient Care Scale) which was developed at Wayne State University in the USA. A simplified version (Wiles 1987) was used for the purpose of assessing the quality of postnatal care and the six topics covered were:

● Staff instructions to the mother;

● Explanation of postnatal care to the mother;

● Pain relief;

● Postnatal exercises;

● Feeding advice;

● Postnatal teaching.

The survey was based on observing a member of staff for a period of two and a half hours with the observer taking on a non-participant role. This meant that the observer could not participate in the care of mothers and babies, except in an emergency situation.

The two main findings of this survey were firstly, that staff did not introduce themselves to the mother, and secondly, that high quality care can be given by very junior staff.

☐ **Suggestion boxes**

Small boxes were made available in each of the four bedded rooms on one postnatal ward and mothers were asked to write down suggestions for improvements in postnatal care (paper and pencils were provided). The main areas of concern were those of linen shortage and poor quality food.

☐ **Conclusions from these three methods of assessing quality**

All three of these methods for assessing the quality of care are valid and should, preferably, be conducted in conjunction with one another and over a period of a year. The results from all three methods pointed towards similar conclusions. Despite the pressure of work and the shortage of staff the quality of postnatal care given by midwifery staff was of an acceptable to high standard. Quality of care was poor, however, in the areas of 'hotel services' (linen, food, cleanliness) – a common problem in the NHS today due to lack of resources.

■ Quality circles

If quality circles are introduced, they could prove to be an integral part of improving postnatal care. As an illustrative example, let us assume that a quality circle has been set up and has identified a specific problem with visiting hours. The selected times for visiting hours in the unit under consideration result in the mothers becoming tired and unable to breastfeed effectively; consequently many are giving up breastfeeding. In addition, women find that they have insufficient time with their partner.

This problem is addressed using the problem solving method outlined on page 147. Analysis and investigation of the problem is performed by carrying out a survey (on both staff and clients) asking them which would be the most convenient visiting hours for their particular needs. Once the results have been analysed, a majority decision can be taken.

As a result of this survey new times for visiting hours can be decided upon. These new visiting hours are then presented to the manager and appropriate personnel with a view to trying out new hours for a period of three months. At the end of this time, the situation needs reviewing as a result of which it may be decided to continue with the new hours, to revert

Figure 9.3   The problem-solving process in action

● Brain storming for a likely problem	Quality circle set up to consider ways of improving postnatal care
● Selecting the most relevant problem	Quality circle identifies problem with visiting hours
● Analysis and investigation of the problem	Surveys are set up to find out what will be the most convenient hours for visiting, for both staff and clients
● Finding a solution for the problem	New visiting hours are drawn up in the light of the survey results
● Implementing the decision	All relevant personnel are informed and new visiting hours are instituted, to be evaluated in three months time

back to the old hours, or to try a further set of new hours. A summary of this process and its relation to straightforward problem solving is given in Fig. 9.3.

■ Assessing postnatal care in the community

The areas chosen for assessing postnatal care in the community will, in some instances, coincide with those assessed in hospital. Areas which interlink are continuity of care, pain relief, postnatal exercises, feeding the baby and postnatal teaching. Those topics specific to the community are more difficult to pinpoint and the following topics are not exhaustive:

● Continuation of breastfeeding;

● Perineal healing, discomfort, problems (for example infection, tight sutures);

● Readmission to hospital, particularly for retained products of conception;

● Attendance at six weeks postnatal examination;

● The use of contraceptives;

● Handover arrangements between community midwife and the health visitor.

There needs to be a flexible approach and good liaison with the client's health visitor. Ideally a time should be arranged when the midwife and health visitor make a joint visit as this would enable a more comprehensive and meaningful handover to take place, thus providing a higher quality of care for the client.

Ideally, the advice which the community midwife gives in the home should be consistent with the advice her client has been given in hospital. If it is necessary to make any alterations, it is essential the community midwife explains to the mother the reason for any change of care. Communication is the essence of good care, so the adequacy and accuracy of the midwife's communications should therefore be beyond question.

In an ideal world the times to monitor the quality of postnatal care would be:

● During the first week postnatally;

● On the 10th postnatal day (at the discharge visit);

● At the 28th day postnatal visit;

● At the six week postnatal examination (a retrospective survey).

■ Assessing and maintaining quality in postnatal care: recommendations for practice

The quality of postnatal care can be assessed but accurate assessment can be complex because different mothers' needs vary so much; this inevitably affects both the methods by which, and the places in which, such care is given. The crux of the matter is that postnatal care has to be 'tailor made' to meet the needs of a particular woman and her family. This can be done by involving the mother in planning and discussing the care, thus providing some measure of continuity.

One might speculate that continuity of care does not need to be given by the same midwife but, perhaps, can be achieved by different midwives giving the same quality of care, thus maintaining standards. The continuity would then relate to the care itself and not to the care giver (see also the chapter by Rosemary Currell on 'The organisation of midwifery care' in the volume in this series on *Antenatal Care*).

An additional way of measuring the quality of care is to monitor complaints. It would be quite easy to analyse complaints and determine what aspects of care are being criticised: midwifery care, domestic or 'hotel' services, personnel or administration.

Ideally there should be a senior group of personnel running a quality assurance programme. This may consist, for example, of a District advisory committee made up of senior managers, a co-ordinating committee at organisational level and standard setting teams at the local level. These local teams should consist of ward staff of mixed grades, no more than six in number. There should also be a mechanism whereby a standard which is written by the ward team is presented to senior management (preferably the Director of Midwifery Services). This standard can then be discussed with other managers, approved, signed and filed with other standards for that specific sphere of practice. Eventually different units between them would have created standards for all aspects of antenatal, intrapartum and post-natal care. The provision of care within these standards should result in a high quality of service being provided for clients and enhanced job satisfaction for midwives.

■ Practice check

☐ Standards

- One way to discover where and when a standard should be set is to think of problem areas you are aware of in your unit. These may include (for example) visiting hours, lack of privacy in the antenatal clinic or labour ward, and the giving of conflicting advice to breastfeeding mothers.

- Using the three tier checklist (structure, process, outcome) set a standard either for a topic of your choice or for one of the above topics.

- Once these standards have been set then use one method for assessing the quality of care to ascertain whether or not these standards are being met.

☐ Assessing quality: questionnaires

- Design a short questionnaire to ascertain whether mothers are receiving conflicting advice about breastfeeding their babies.

- If the advice is conflicting, your questionnaire should enable you to discover the reason.

- It should be borne in mind that questionnaires involving clients will have to be approved by the Ethics Committee.

☐ Assessing quality: peer observation

- Devise a simple scoring system for the standard of care you would expect from a midwife carrying out postnatal observations.

- One midwife is to observe a peer midwife for up to two hours and then score according to your plan. Obviously a very low score would indicate cause for concern.

☐ **Assessing quality: suggestion box**

- Leave an empty box (accompanied by paper and pencils) and ask the mothers to write down one or two suggestions for improvements to postnatal care.

- Analyse the suggestions and inform appropriate personnel as and when necessary.

☐ **Quality circles**

- Form a group of between four and six staff. Prioritise the problems in the clinical area and select one problem to work on using the problem solving approach.

☐ **Monitoring quality**

- What areas of postnatal care would you monitor to ensure a high quality of care in hospital or in the community?

■ References

All Wales Nurse Manpower Planning Committee (Midwifery Sub-group) 1986 Standards of postnatal care. HMSO, London

Christie H, O'Reilly M 1984 Quality circles. Nursing Mirror   158 (6): 16–19

Dunne L M 1986 Defining quality assurance practice. Professional Nurse   1 (11): 47

Hyde P 1984 Quality circles 1. Something for everyone. Nursing Times   80 (48): 49–50

Kitson A Steps to setting achievable nursing standards. Unpublished Standards of Care project, RCN, London

Maternity Services Advisory Committee 1985 Maternity care in action. Part III, Care of mother and baby. HMSO, London

Nunnerley R 1988 Assessing the quality of postnatal care in hospital. Parjon

Nursing Standard 1987 Supplement: In pursuit of excellence. Volume 2   (10): 2–15

Ray G 1986 Postnatal care. Johnson & Johnson Baby Newsline   42 (Autumn)

Samuel J, Balch B 1985 Maternity care in action part III: care of mother and baby. Midwives Chronicle 98 (1169): 161–62
United Kingdom Central Council 1986 Midwives' Rules and Code of Practice and Code of Professional Conduct: 144. UKCC, London
Wiles A 1987 Quality of patient care scale. In Pearson A (ed) Nursing quality measurement: quality assurance methods for peer review. John Wiley, Chichester

■ Suggested further reading

Ball J 1989 Postnatal care and adjustment to motherhood. In Robinson S, Thomson A (eds) Midwives, research and childbirth. Chapman and Hall, London
Hughes D J F, Goldstone L A 1989 Frameworks for midwifery care in Great Britain: an exploration of quality assurance. Midwifery 5 (4): 163–71
Kitson A 1986 Indicators of quality in nursing care: an alternative approach. Journal of Advanced Nursing 11: 133–44
Kitson A 1989 A framework for quality: a patient centered approach to quality assurance in health care. Scutari Press, Harrow
Lorentzon M 1987 Quality in nursing – the state of the art. Senior Nurse 7 (6): 11–12
Maternity Services Advisory Committee 1985 Maternity care in action. Part III, Care of mother and baby. HMSO, London
Pearson A 1987 Nursing quality measurement: quality assurance methods for peer review. John Wiley, Chichester
Royal College of Midwives 1987 RCM Statement 'Towards a healthy nation': a policy for the maternity services. Midwives Chronicle 100 (1194): 218
Wilson C R M 1989 Hospital-wide quality assurance. W B Saunders, Philadelphia, Toronto

■ Appendix to Chapter 9: Quality assurance in postnatal care

☐ 1. Staff questionnaire: survey on the quality of postnatal care

I am a midwifery manager undertaking studies at the Thames Polytechnic for the postgraduate course entitled 'Diploma in Management Studies' (Health Services) CNAA.

I am doing some research into the quality of postnatal care in hospital as part of my studies and I hope you will be able to help me by answering the following questionnaire.

WARD PROFILE

1. No. of available postnatal beds   ....

2. No. of occupied postnatal beds   ....

3. Total no. of staff on duty during a 24-hour period
   a) Early shift   ....
   b) Late shift   ....
   c) Night duty   ....

4. What were the grades of staff on:
   (Please state numbers of appropriate grades
   alongside tick e.g. ☑2)

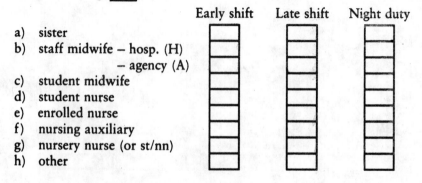

	Early shift	Late shift	Night duty
a) sister			
b) staff midwife – hosp. (H)			
– agency (A)			
c) student midwife			
d) student nurse			
e) enrolled nurse			
f) nursing auxiliary			
g) nursery nurse (or st/nn)			
h) other			

POSTNATAL CARE

	YES	NO

5. a) Do you involve the mother in planning her postnatal care? ☐ ☐

    b) If yes, please explain briefly

    ....

    ....

6. What standard of postnatal care do you think your ward staff
    give to the mothers?

    a) excellent ☐
    b) good ☐
    c) adequate ☐
    d) minimal but safe ☐

    Comments: ....

	YES	NO

7. a) Do you have any form of continuity of care? ☐ ☐

    b) If yes, please elaborate briefly

    ....

	YES	NO

8. a) Do you involve the partner with the postnatal care of the ☐ ☐
    baby?

    b) If no, please give details/reasons

    ....

    ....

FEEDING ADVICE

9. a) Has any mother ever said to you or your staff that she has YES   NO
    received conflicting advice as to how to feed her baby?   ☐   ☐

    b) If yes, how have you dealt with the situation?

    ....

    ....

POSTNATAL TEACHING

10. Do you teach/show mothers (particularly first time) any of the
    following baby care topics before they go home

	YES	NO
a) bathing a baby	☐	☐
b) folding a nappy		
c) making up a feed and sterilizing equipment		
d) cord care		
e) other topic (state)		

    ....

    ....

11. If no to any of the above questions is it for any of the
    following reasons?

                                                                                  YES   NO

    a) mother has previous children
    b) mother did not wish to be shown
    c) staff did not have time
    d) other (specify)

    ....
    ....

                                                                                YES   NO

12. Do you ever have a shortage of linen?

13. If yes, is

    a) disposable linen used?
    b) mother asked to bring in own bed linen?
    c) mother asked to bring in baby linen?

VISITING HOURS

14. What are your maternity unit's visiting hours?

    Morning   from . . . . . . to . . . . . .
    Afternoon from . . . . . . to . . . . . .
    Evening   from . . . . . . to . . . . . .

15. Do they in any way hinder   YES   NO

    a) giving care to the mothers or baby?
    b) the mother from feeding her baby?
    c) the mother from resting?
    d) the mother from eating her meals?

16. If yes, to any of the above, state what has been done to
    improve the situation?

    ....
    ....

17. State 2 or 3 factors which you feel prevent you from giving the
    standard of postnatal care you would like to give to each
    mother/baby

    a) ....
    b) ....
    c) ....

18. Additional comments:

Thank you for sparing your valuable time in answering this questionnaire.

Rowan Nunnerley, November 1987

☐ **2. Mothers' questionnaire: survey on the quality of postnatal care**

I am a midwifery manager undertaking studies at the Thames Polytechnic for the postgraduate course entitled 'Diploma in Management Studies' (Health Services) CNAA.

I am doing some research into the quality of postnatal care in hospital as part of my studies and hope that you will be able to help me by answering the following questionnaire.

DELIVERY/CHILDREN   TICK BOX/ES

1. a) How was your baby born?

                                                Normally ☐
           Forceps ☐
           Breech ☐
           Ventouse ☐
           Caesarean ☐
           Twins ☐

   b) How many days ago was your baby born   ....

                                        YES   NO

   c) Is this your first baby   ☐   ☐

   d) If no, how many children have you had before   ....

ARRIVAL ON THE POSTNATAL WARD

2. When you arrived on the postnatal ward from delivery suite, were you:

                                        YES   NO

   a) Welcomed?   ☐   ☐
   b) Shown/told where bathroom and toilets were situated?   ☐   ☐
   c) Introduced to other mothers in room/ward?   ☐   ☐
   d) Offered a drink or jug of water?   ☐   ☐
   e) Shown/told where to put suitcase and belongings?   ☐   ☐

DAILY CARE

                                        YES   NO

3. a) Do you ever have a choice in planning care for yourself   ☐   ☐
      and your baby with the midwifery staff looking after you?
   b) If yes please give brief details

   ....
   ....

                                        YES   NO

4. Has the midwife explained why you and your baby are   ☐   ☐
   examined each day?

5. Who out of the following staff examines

    YOU   YOUR BABY

    a) midwife
    b) student midwife
    c) student nurse
    d) enrolled nurse
    e) nursing auxiliary
    f) nursery nurse/student nursery nurse
    g) don't know

6. When you and your baby are examined each day does
    the same person see

    YOU   YOUR BABY

    a) every day
    b) most days
    c) occasional days
    d) one day only

PAIN RELIEF

7. If you have pain or discomfort does a midwife/nurse
    come to see you within

    a) a few minutes?
    b) 5–10 minutes?
    c) 10–15 minutes?
    d) 15–30 minutes?
    e) 30 minutes or more?

8. If you ask for pain relief is it given to you within

    a) a few minutes?
    b) 5–10 minutes?
    c) 10–15 minutes?
    d) 30 minutes or more?

POSTNATAL EXERCISES

9. Have you been taught or shown how to do postnatal
    exercises?

    YES   NO

10. If yes, who taught you?

    a) midwife
    b) physiotherapist
    c) student midwife
    d) other staff

11. Do you understand why it is important to do postnatal exercises?

    YES ☐   NO ☐

12. Have you been given a leaflet of instructions about postnatal exercises?

    YES ☐   NO ☐

FEEDING YOUR BABY

13. Are you:

    YES   NO

    a) Breastfeeding? ☐ ☐

    b) Bottle feeding? ☐ ☐

14. Is the advice about feeding your baby

    a) always the same ☐

    b) sometimes the same ☐

    c) never the same ☐

15. a) Has the advice ever been conflicting/confusing

    YES ☐   NO ☐

    b) If yes please give further details

    ....

    ....

    ....

LINEN

16. Were you asked to bring any of the following into hospital with you?

    a) nappies ☐

    b) baby towels ☐

    c) baby clothes ☐

    d) other items ....

    ....

17. Have disposable (paper) cot sheets or baby clothes ever been used because the ward had run out of linen?

    YES ☐   NO ☐

18. Has soiled linen been kept on *your* bed because the ward had run out of linen?

    YES ☐   NO ☐

POSTNATAL TEACHING

19. Which of the following babycare topics have been taught
    on the ward?
    a) bathing your baby
    b) folding a nappy
    c) making up a bottle feed and sterilising
       equipment
    d) care of baby's cord
    e) other topics (state)

    ....
    ....

                                                                    YES   NO
20. Has your partner been involved in caring for your baby?   ☐   ☐

21. If no, what is the reason?
    a) working
    b) preferred not to be involved
    c) frightened
    d) staff did not encourage him
    e) other reason (state)

    ....
    ....

VISITING HOURS

22. What are the visiting hours?

    Morning   From . . . . .   To . . . . . .
    Afternoon   From . . . . . .   To . . . . . .
    Evening   From . . . . . .   To . . . . . .

23. Do the visiting hours prevent you from
                                                    YES   NO
    a) resting?
    b) having time for yourself?
    c) being alone with your partner?
    d) feeding your baby?
    e) eating your own meals?

24. Additional comments you may like to make about your
    care in the postnatal ward

Thank your for sparing your valuable time to complete this questionnaire.

Rowan Nunnerley, November 1987

☐ **Peer observation survey**

MOTHER:	POSTNATAL TOPICS	
A Introductions Staff code/s:		
	Had the midwife/nurse introduced herself to the mother by giving	Tick one box
1.	(All three) Her name, staff grade, and how long she will be looking after mother	☐
2.	(Two out of three) Name/staff grade, *or* Staff grade/how long she will be looking after mother *or* Name/how long she will be looking after mother	☐
3.	(One out of the three) Name or staff grade or how long she will be looking after mother	☐
4.	Greeting only (e.g. Hello)	☐
5.	No introduction of herself at all	☐
B Explanation of care Staff code/s:		
	When care was given to the mother and/or baby did the midwife/nurse	Tick boxes
1.	Explain exactly what she was doing	☐
2.	Give the reason why she was doing it	☐
3.	Allow the mother to help plan the day's care	☐
4.	Listen to the mother's questions	☐
5.	Answer the questions to the mother's satisfaction	☐

MOTHER:	POSTNATAL TOPICS	(cont.)

C Pain Relief   Staff code/s:

	Circle YES/NO
Was pain relief required?	
If yes, did the midwife or nurse come and give the pain relief to the mother within	Tick one box
i) A few minutes	☐
ii) 5–10 minutes	☐
iii) 10–15 minutes	☐
iv) 15–30 minutes	☐

D Postnatal exercises   Staff code/s:

	'✓'(Yes) 'X'(No)
i) Had postnatal exercises been discussed?	☐
ii) Had postnatal exercises been shown or taught?	☐
iii) Had a leaflet of instructions been given to the mother?	☐
iv) Were questions/worries dealt with? (If none write 'N' in box)	☐
v) Did the mother understand the importance of doing postnatal exercises?	☐

E Feeding advice   Staff code/s:

Tick one box	
Method of feeding: Breast	☐
Bottle	☐
Both	☐
Was any advice given to mother regarding feeding her baby? If YES	Circle YES/NO
	Tick one box
i) Was advice given with explanation and recorded in 'COMB' chart?	☐
ii) Was advice given with explanation but not recorded in 'COMB' chart? *or* Was advice given without explanation but recorded in 'COMB' chart?	☐
iii) Was the advice given without explanation and without recording in 'COMB' chart?	☐
('COMB' – Care Of Mothers and Babies)	

MOTHER:	POSTNATAL TOPICS	(cont.)

F Postnatal teaching Staff code/s:

Had/Did any postnatal teaching take place during
2 hour period? YES/NO
  If YES what was the topic ....
  If NO give reason ....
....

(If teaching not done during 2 hour observation period please ask the
mother the following questions related to any other postnatal teaching)

		VW	W	S	P
i)	Did the midwife/nurse teach	4	3	2	1
ii)	How did the mother understand what was taught	4	3	2	1
iii)	Did the midwife/nurse allow the mother to ask questions		Circle YES/NO		
iv)	If YES, how did the midwife or nurse answer them	4	3	2	1

(VW = Very well; W = Well; S = Satisfactorily; P = Poorly)

Comments from observer:

Comments from mother given to observer:

☐ **Peer observation survey: quality of care results**

MOTHER	A	B	C	D	E	F	Total Score
Topic Total							Overall Total
% Topic Total							Overall %

Index

questions:
  antenatal booking interview 1.47, 52
  antenatal education 1.97–8
Quetelet Index 1.4, 14

reflexology 2.106
Rescue Remedy 2.106
retardation of intrauterine growth
    1.111
risk, and place of birth 2.2–5
roles 1.127–8
rooting 3.21, 70
Royal College of Midwives:
  and antenatal booking 1.44, 48
  and antenatal education 1.91–2
  and breastfeeding preparation 1.68
  and place of birth 2.17–18
rubella 1.10–11
rupture of membranes see membranes

SAFTA 3.124
salt baths, postnatal 3.4–5, 13
SANDS 3.119, 124
schools, health education in 3.137–8
screening, health, preconception
    1.9–11
second stage of labour 2.122–33
  duration of 2.123–4
  onset of 2.123
  position for 2.124–5, 132
  prevention of perineal trauma
    2.126–31, 132
  pushing 2.125–6, 132
self-concept 1.127
'sensitive period' for attachment 3.63,
    65
sex, resumption after birth 3.12
Sexual Offences Act (1956) 3.130
shared care 1.22, 29, 32–3
  and analgesia 2.11
  and multiple births 1.137, 140, 142
shaving, perineum 2.32, 38
shells, breast 1.66–7
Short Report (1980) 1.25, 2.13
Sighthill scheme 1.28, 48
silver nitrate 3.20–1
silver sulphadiazine 3.88
smiling, neonate 3.72
smoking see tobacco
Social Services Committee (1980) 2.9
sophrology 2.109–10
special care baby units (SCBUs)
    3.98–101
  see also transitional care

specificity theory of pain 2.72–3
spontaneous delivery 2.122–33
  duration of second stage 2.123–4
  onset of second stage 2.123
  position 2.124–5, 132
  prevention of perineal trauma
    2.126–31, 132
  pushing 2.125–6, 132
standards of care 3.145–6, 148–9
Staphylococcus 3.86–8
stillbirth 3.112–15, 117–19
Stillbirth and Neonatal Death
    Association (SANDS) 3.119,
    124
stomach, emptying in labour 2.60, 65–6
stress:
  and child abuse 3.130
  and nutrition in labour 2.60
  postnatal 3.50–1, 53, 130
  preconception 1.7–8
  pregnancy 1.124, 129
structure criteria 3.146, 150
subfertility 1.9, 14
'summation' theory of pain 2.74
supplementary feeding, neonate 3.30,
    36
sutures, perineal repair 2.130–1, 132
Syntometrine 2.139

TAMBA 1.139, 143–4, 3.124
teaching skills, antenatal education
    1.88
team midwifery 1.30
technology:
  fetal heart monitoring 2.26–7, 43,
    46–8
  ultrasound (q.v.) 1.105–17
  see also intervention in labour
teenage mothers 3.125–39
  and adoption 3.133–4
  antenatal care 3.131–2, 138
  benefits and resources available
    3.129–30, 134
  health education in schools 3.137–8
  medical and obstetric risks 3.131–2
  mother's education 3.135
  parenthood education 3.135–7
  social factors 3.126–30
  and termination 3.126–7, 133
temperature control, transitional care
    3.103
termination of pregnancy 3.111–12
  teenage mothers 3.126–7, 133
test weighing 3.32–3, 36